And Not to Yield

Marie L. Reed

Monique
Thank you for
allowing me to share
My Story
Marie

First Edition – February 2013

ISBN
978-1-4602-0818-2 (Hardcover)
978-1-4602-0816-8 (Paperback)
978-1-4602-0817-5 (eBook)

Rae Anne Lawrason
Illustrations and artwork

Editors: Jen Hiuser of Elequent Editing
Phyllis Kozak and Stephanie Wilson

Janice Godbout
Photograph of Jarryd and Cole fishing on front cover

Produced by:

FriesenPress
Suite 300 – 852 Fort Street
Victoria, BC, Canada V8W 1H8

www.friesenpress.com

Distributed to the trade by The Ingram Book Company

Dedication

To my dear sweet boys Jarryd and Cole, whom I love with all my heart.

Thank you for your belief and encouragement.

I hope this book gives my children the opportunity to know each family member in heaven, and to understand how blessed we are to have had these remarkable people in our lives, even if only for a short while.

Author's Message

We get so caught up in where we're headed we often forget to enjoy the steps that brought us there in the first place.

Fortunately, I have two beautiful young boys who make me pay attention! Though I am always there for them, it isn't always quality time. I thought, if I could only slow down long enough to really enjoy them and truly engage in what they are saying.

During all of this they were crying out for help. Oh, it was loud and clear, but I felt that I didn't know how to help them. I often didn't know what to say. I couldn't in all honesty tell them that Daddy was going to be all right, because I didn't know that for certain. I didn't want them to hold me to any promises I couldn't keep. After all, saying it was going to be all right may have made me a liar.

Instead, I decided to simply be there for them and to remain positive. Some people asked if I was in denial. I responded by saying that I didn't know what they were talking about, for I truly believed that God would take care of everything. I didn't think that the only possible outcome was good, but I did know that God would take care of everything, no matter the outcome. That way I could accept this in my heart and stay strong for Jarryd and Cole.

My sister-in-law Janice took a snapshot of my boys while I was at the hospital with Shawn. This photograph captures the calmness of their little bodies as they stand side by side casting into the river. The colours are magical! A Monet painting is the only thing that could touch this kind of beauty: water colours reflecting the vibrant autumn bouquet surrounding them. They are unaware that the picture is being taken, because they are entirely absorbed in that moment.

Aren't children *amazing*? They still have the ability to grab hold of moments and devour every delectable morsel. When do adults lose this ability? Maybe it is our fast-paced lives or our inability to slow down long enough to pay attention. I remember getting that photograph from Janice and immediately wanting it framed. I was sorry that I had missed it. I had missed being there at that moment and I had missed slowing down often enough to feel fully present in my childrens' lives.

If all of this has taught me anything, I have learned to examine from different angles. I compare it to teaching. If your students don't understand something one way, you teach it differently – from another angle or perspective.

I could have merely viewed the photograph as just another snapshot of my children, as I do have thousands, but for some reason this image really stood out. The message was staring me in the face – they were frozen in the moment – and this was captured on film. I was missing the beauty in life, in nature, and in them. I needed to breathe in deeply, capture the aroma and see that bouquet of colours as a metaphor for life. Stop and smell the flowers right under my nose and linger in their essence; let them consume me.

This is when I knew I had to write this book. The day we found out about my husband's cancer was definitely the day our whole world "turned on a dime". We were on top of the world one minute and crushed beneath it the next. This made me freeze in my tracks and realize all I took for granted. The single photograph on the cover of this book, gave me insight. My two innocent boys, captured in a moment, brought me inspiration! It is my hope that after reading my book, you may come to realize,

Life will pass you by if you don't pay attention.

Chapter One

Lexi

Comfort can be found in the most unexpected places. When I cuddled up to Lexi, I was at peace. She was my sanity in a crazy world and also a soothing resting place for my weary head. Her velvet fur, sweet puppy smell, and big sad eyes left me feeling innocent. I could retreat to a place where nothing could hurt me – a momentary refuge into complete protection and unconditional love.

I remember the day we picked her out…after I swore I didn't want a pooping, sleeping, eating machine. But, Shawn and the boys were relentless and certain Mom would be mere putty in their hands; unable to resist their pleas.

Shawn was the master! He meticulously researched, surfing the internet for the best prices, meanwhile making sure to show me pictures of every adorable puppy he found. Oh, he was good, and after weeks passed, I finally agreed to meet with a breeder from Hull, Quebec, to check out two fourteen weekold, female Bullmastiff pups.

Next to her sister, Lexi looked hilarious with those overgrown paws and pitiful face. They sat side by side, colourful leashes draped around their necks, and their wrinkled heads slightly tilted to one side as if to say "See how cute I am? You want to adopt me. Really you do!"

The first words out of my mouth were, "Awwww...aren't they cute!"

Because Hull, Quebec was three hours away from our home, the breeder agreed to meet in a parking lot in Ottawa so that we could view his two remaining female pups. The boys and I instantly noticed a bite mark forming a fresh scab on the head of the white pup. Cole, being five years old at the time, rudely pointed at her and said, "Oooh Mommy, that one looks ugly!" I gently pushed his hand down, feeling a little embarrassed.

We joked later, remarking on how our Lexi had most definitely mauled her sister so that she would look ugly and not be adopted that day. But, truth be told, Lexi was fawn-coloured, while her sister was white. This gave her a definite advantage, for we had already set our hearts on a fawn coloured pup. Shawn handed the guy an envelope containing a cool grand and I remember feeling as if we had just completed a drug deal. But apparently, this was cheap for a Bullmastiff.

Reluctant to leave her sister, Lexi wasn't sure about this whole deal of belonging to our family and she especially wasn't keen about getting into a strange vehicle. She sat back on her haunches, turning her twenty-five pound frame into dead weight, and we ended up having to hoist her with that big wrinkled head into the backseat of our car.

As we drove away, I became thoroughly disgusted about the money that had exchanged hands, and began complaining, "I have never paid for a dog in my life!" I continued to grumble, "On the farm, we always had mutts or Heinz 57's. None of this purebred, high falutin, registered malarkey." Then, I stopped myself in mid-thought, thinking how much I sounded like my parents, and a little smile crept across my face.

Hunkering down and shaking in the backseat, nerves (and perhaps fear) got the better of Lexi. We had just stopped at Taco Bell for some nice, greasy tacos, and as soon as we got the food in the car Lexi decided to leave a big old mushy poop on the back seat. Thank goodness the seats were leather, and we were able to pull into a gas station to wipe them down. But, considering it was a hot day, the lingering stench soon filtered into the front seat.

Needless to say, the tacos were no longer appealing and we pulled over and tossed them into the garbage.

The ribbing began. My sons couldn't wait to mock me, as they more-or-less repeated the first words out of my mouth when I saw Lexi and her sister sitting on that curb: "Awww, aren't they cute!"

Shawn had wanted a Bullmastiff since he was a child. While growing up, he had a friend who owned one and he would tell me how they were gentle giants. He reminisced about how he and Brutis (his friend's Mastiff) would wrestle. Shawn would grab Brutis' enormous head in both hands, jostling him about, slapping his sloppy jowls, and Brutis would play ever so gently. Shawn told me that although Brutis looked like he could swallow him whole, he was a big marshmallow. You see, Bullmastiffs were originally bred to search out and stop poachers, but somewhere along the way they had become house pets. They are known to jump on intruders, knocking them to the ground, while growling, and exposing their ferocious teeth. Meanwhile, drool drips from their gaping lips. *Very attractive*! They don't attack, but rather hold the unsuspecting shmuck down until someone pulls their one hundred fifty to two hundred pound frame from the victim's chest.

This is what they are known for, but anyone who owns a Bullmastiff knows that they are kindhearted, affectionate creatures. You definitely want to stay on their good side, but they will never attack without cause. They typically bond to one person and become a loyal companion.

From that day on, it became apparent that Lexi was *my dog* – go figure!

It's funny, when you believe there is something you don't want or need, and that very thing becomes your lifeline. That is what Lexi became – my wrinkle-headed, velvet-eared, droopy-lipped confidant – and essentially my *lifeline*.

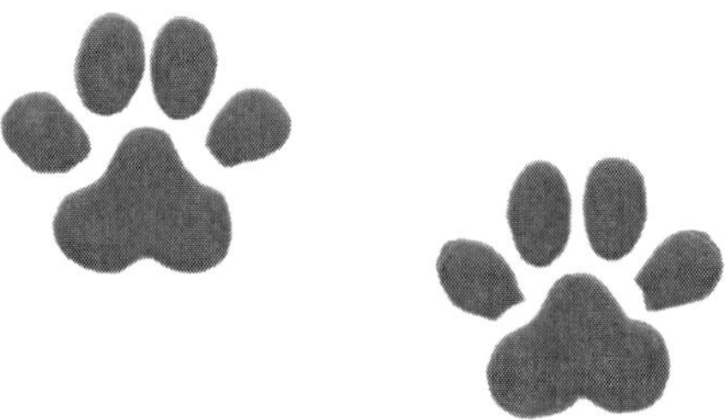

And yes, Cole, my youngest son still loves to tease me, and reminds me almost daily how *I didn't want a dog*.

When I hugged Lexi, everything was okay. I felt an inner peace, even though my world was about to come tumbling down around me.

* * * * *

Shawn and I cruised down the pavement in our little WRX sports car, feeling the warmth of the sun flood across the windscreen and through the open sunroof. As we entered the hospital's emergency entrance, we saw several patients standing outside attached to IV machines and smoking cigarettes. It was unspoken, but I knew we were both thinking how lucky we were not to be one of these poor people – weak with illness and addicted to nicotine. We almost felt guilty, seeming to not have a care in the world.

In fact, I remember Shawn saying how lucky he felt as he squeezed my hand. He told me how much he loved our life together. I had never met anyone so passionate about life. He knew how to express his exact feelings at any moment and he made me feel, like I was the most beautiful woman alive.

We parked the car, jumped out, and went bounding up the stairs to where the medical offices were located. We were running late for our appointment and giggling like school children; racing up to the elevator and half running down the hallway. We still had goofy grins on our faces as Dr. Greggor stepped out of his office. We began to apologize for our tardiness, but Dr. Greggor showed little concern, as he was preoccupied. I thought his behaviour was odd, and felt especially uncomfortable by the way he said, "Oh…you brought your wife."

Shawn introduced me and we shook hands. Dr. Greggor motioned for us to enter his office and closed the door behind us.

Earlier in the week, Shawn had been in for some tests to determine why his ulcers were not improving. We were almost certain that his ulcers must have been perforated.

Barely making eye contact, Dr. Greggor simply slid the colour photographs across the table to explain the findings of the colonoscopy. I wasn't familiar with what I was looking at. They were definitely pictures of a stomach, but there appeared to be another organ, and this organ was black. Somewhat bewildered, Shawn began to ask a few questions. Dr. Greggor interrupted stating, "This is cancer."

What he said after that was inaudible, like the disorientation that occurs from a heat wave in the desert. All of my senses shut down and there was this deafening stillness in the room. I stared in disbelief while Shawn began to sob. I felt ridiculous, because I was holding him, comforting him, but I was paralyzed. We could see the grief in Dr. Greggor's eyes. He was about the same age as we were, and had two small children of his own. He could barely articulate his next words. He wouldn't give

Shawn any definitive answers about the severity of the cancer, but by his somber demeanor, I knew it wasn't good.

Chapter Two

Frozen

When you find out your life will be changed forever, things happen very quickly. I walked around in a fog – motoring along like a programmed robot.

Must feed kids

Must fold laundry

Must remember to keep appointments

It was second nature to just forge ahead and get things done. I think I was simply on autopilot. No time to think. Just do what was needed.

Because the military had transferred Shawn to Ontario and most of our family was spread across Canada and the United States, I corresponded regularly by email.

August 9, 2007

Dear Family and Friends,

Jarryd and Cole, like most of us, are trying to figure out what is going on. If you can imagine how confused we adults are, you can imagine how difficult this is for their little minds to grasp. At first we didn't want to scare them with the 'C' word because they've lost both of their grandpas to this horrible thing, so instead we told them that Daddy had to go for a very important surgery on his stomach and we left it at that. As time went on, we knew that the word would slip and they would wonder why we hadn't told them the truth. We didn't want to lose their trust, so we decided it was best to sit them down and tell them about the cancer, but assure them that this one was curable. Jarryd didn't know how to react, so instead, he pretended to hyperventilate – at least I thought he was pretending. I told him that there was no correct way in which to react, and that feeling numb or frozen was also a reaction. This I knew from firsthand experience. I explained that when the doctor told me, I sat there as if a truck had hit me in the face. Cole didn't react much because he didn't understand anything we were saying, and two minutes later, he was joking around. That was okay too, because better that than what we are all going through.

Love Marie

Probably one of the hardest phone calls I had to make was to Jasmine and Amber, Shawn's daughters from his first marriage. They lived in Florida with their mother. We had been there on vacation just a few weeks prior, before the news when life was simple.

It was fifteen year old Amber who answered.

Her sweet voice was on the phone. "Hello," she said.

"Hi Amber, it's Marie calling."

"Hi Marie, how are you?" she inquired.

I hadn't the slightest idea how I would tell her. Her voice was cheery and carefree – the last thing I wanted, was to drop this bombshell on her. I gathered my strength – I certainly didn't want her and her sister to find out in an email, or worse, to hear about it from someone else. *I was shaking now.*

I drew a deep breath. "Amber, you know how your dad was having a hard time eating when we were in Florida?"

"Yes," she replied.

"He went for some tests on his stomach when we got back. The doctor couldn't understand why his ulcers were not getting better with the medication he was taking."

"Is he…*okay*?" She asked tentatively.

I paused, gathering my strength. "Amber, they found cancer."

The line went painfully silent.

I continued, "He needs an operation to remove the cancer."

She was crying now. "Oh Marie – *that is so terrible*!"

"Amber, this one is curable. Try not to worry. Could you please tell Jasmine and your mom for me?"

"Yes." Her voice was barely audible. "Of course I will Marie."

"Take care sweetie." My voice was breaking now. "I am so sorry I had to give you this news."

Chapter Three

Joy in the Chaos

Between hospital visits, Lexi was brand new and needed to be trained. She didn't fit into those paws. It was hilarious how she would leap off the deck and try to find her footing with those big old moccasins flailing around. It was as if her feet were four weighted baseball bats and she had to coordinate them to work in sync. She would jump off the deck, legs flailing, and then do a face plant with her ears flying up in the air. Eventually, gravity would pull her ears back down to earth.

She brought us plenty of joy amidst the chaos.

She had us laughing at times when we felt guilty laughing. She brought happiness when we thought we would never feel happiness again. It was as though we would feel normal for a fleeting moment and then feel guilty that we had actually smiled at a time of such heartbreak. In spite of, multiple hospital visits and the devastating prognosis, Lexi brought joy into our lives. Call it distraction or comic relief. She was a *blessing*.

Sometimes we had to leave Lexi at home with Nana or in her kennel.

I cursed the idiotic idea of *getting a dog at this time*.

I could still hear Shawn's pleas, "Please Marie, she's what I have always wanted, and when I'm better I promise to walk her every day!" yatta yatta yatta

What was I thinking?

While we were away for hours at a time, Lexi would sometimes rebel by leaving nice juicy gifts around the house. The only thing is, they didn't smell pretty and they definitely weren't wrapped with pretty bows. I cursed that dog, and would begin yelling. But then, I'd look at that big wrinkled head and those sad eyes, and would instantly melt.

When we first got her, I took a picture of Shawn holding Lexi in his arms, kissing that big head of hers with her enormous paws draped over his arm. He was looking directly into the camera with his soft blue eyes, like a big kid who had just unwrapped the present of his dreams. Later, I gave each of the boys a framed photo of this picture to keep in their rooms. Even now, they still fall asleep while looking into their Dad`s eyes and talking with him at great lengths. That in itself is a *gift*.

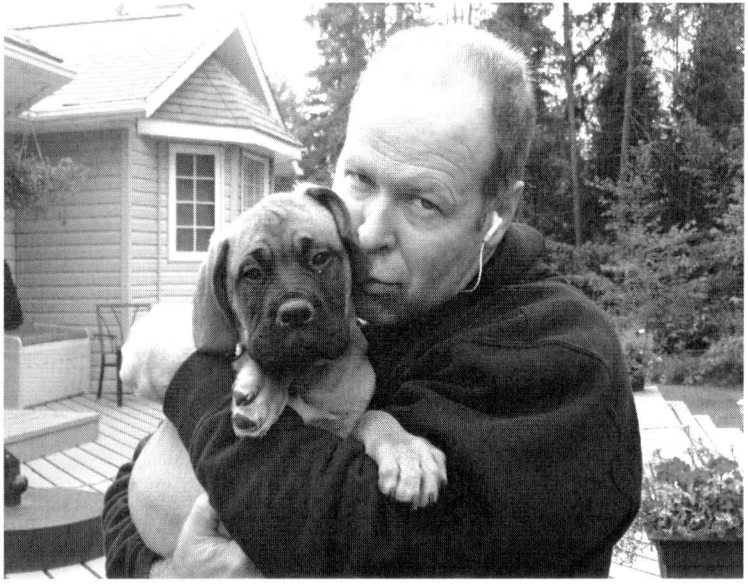

Lexi made Shawn happy. She gave him something to look forward to. I would have given anything to take away some of his sadness and fear. I could not imagine how difficult it must have been for him to not know how much time he had left. It was a malicious joke! Here was a man who appeared perfectly healthy, yet he was *dying*. I tried to wrap my head around it, but it was unfathomable on every level. It was as though Satan himself was cruelly pointing his foreboding finger, staring Shawn square in the face with a wretched laugh, and damning him to endure a sentence equal to the fires of hell.

What was most incomprehensible to me was how undeserving Shawn was of this sentence. He had lived a clean life. By this, I am simply saying, he was a good person. He had dedicated his life to helping others. He served in the Canadian military, and had always asserted how he was there 'to help and not to harm'. In fact, he had chosen the medical profession, starting as a nurse practitioner/paramedic and continuing on to train as a Biomedical Engineer. This meant that he fixed hospital equipment from simple IV machines to highly technical equipment such as MRI machines and CT scanners. His hopes were to serve his remaining five years in the military, receive a pension, and then find a respectable job in a local hospital. This way, he would no longer have to leave his family to serve in countries halfway around the world.

Growing up, his life hadn't been easy. He was raised in an inner-city suburb of Toronto. His dad left him, his sister, and his mother when Shawn was only four years old. His mother finished her nursing training and worked as much as she could to provide a good life for her children. But between work and daycare, she didn't bring in much pay, so they had to rely on government assistance.

Shawn worked extremely hard for everything he had. He took pride in the fact that he had escaped the potential life he could have fallen into. Many of the kids he had grown up with dropped out of school and turned to a life of drugs or crime. But, Shawn worked two jobs which enabled him to enroll in a private high school. Later, he furthered his education, by achieving a degree in architecture at Humber College. Charismatic and with a gift for leadership, Shawn ran for President of the Student's Union. With his boyish charm and well-kept promises, he easily won the support of his fellow students. He was a man of his word and did well by his peers. After graduating from college, he began working in the field of architecture, but decided he couldn't be confined to an office, and signed up with the Canadian Forces, originally as an engineer.

To listen to Shawn, you would swear he had lived three lifetimes. I had never known anyone who pushed themselves this hard. He had packed so much education and life experiences into his forty-two years. He was remarkable to listen to, and as he spoke, I realized how little I had lived in comparison. But I also knew how fortunate I was not to have endured the many hardships that came with his tumultuous life.

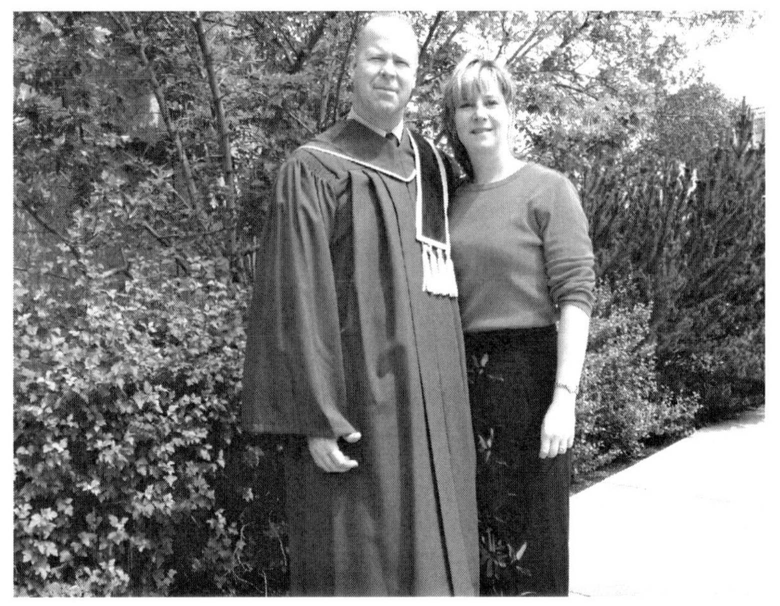

Graduating from the Northern Alberta Institute Of Technology in 2004 as a Biomedical Engineer.

Chapter Four

The Day of Miracles

When one mysterious event occurs in a day, you may or may not pay attention. But when several unexplainable events unfold, you are forced to take notice.

Shawn had just undergone his first surgery and was recuperating in the recovery room. We were now able to see him, and I had no idea what to expect. I was in a half-walk, half-run down a hallway that seemed to have no end, while my thoughts weighed heavily. *I knew things would never be the same.*

There he was, my beautiful husband, lying on a stretcher. He was coherent, even alert, which surprised me. I grabbed his hand and held it in mine while I fought back tears.

He said, "I did it!"

"You certainly did!"

"This is my second chance," he added.

"Yes it is. I am so proud of you. Shawn, I love you so much!"

"God, how I love you. You are the girl of my dreams."

I smiled reassuringly, "You rest now and I will see you in a little while."

And I kissed his lips, paying attention to every detail – how they felt pressed to mine, the warmth, the fullness, the wetness – drinking it all in. These lips I had kissed a thousand times.

As I walked out of the room, I had mixed feelings of joy and sadness. I felt blessed that he had made it through the surgery, but I also knew that his life would be forever altered.

The relief I felt a moment ago, was replaced with an uncontrollable rage. It seemed to come out of nowhere.

Why him? A man who serves his country – a man who puts others before himself… a man who loves his family dearly and who grew up with so much pain. Why him, God? Why? My face felt flush, as the hot tears came in droves, streaking my cheeks with every ounce of bitterness. I wanted to punch something real hard, to let go of the anger I felt inside.

Next came the feeling of utter defeat – the vulnerability you experience when you have no control over your life. When life kicks you in the gut, and you have no choice but to just take it. The raw meat of your insides are rolled over and exposed to the world. Like a beaten dog, you have absolutely no recourse.

Shawn was transferred to a recovery ward with twenty-four hour care. His mother and I took turns staying with him. He was scared. I could see it in his eyes, but he was attempting to be incredibly brave. He had such a high threshold for pain. They had him hopped up on all kinds of pain medication, but nothing was taking the edge off. The nurses and doctors were baffled, and started performing ice tests to see if he could feel pain at his incision. That is when they discovered that the epidural had not taken. Instead, they had frozen the wrong side of his body. This meant he had come out of surgery without any freezing over the surgical site. I felt sick inside, now realizing how much he must have endured once the anesthetic wore off.

I was fuming! Was this some sort of Gong Show? Hadn't Shawn been through enough? But then, I remembered how this was a training hospital, and how the anesthesiologist explained that a resident would be administering the epidural under her supervision. How could I have let that happen? I should have demanded that the physician give the epidural!

As if this wasn't enough, when the physiotherapist entered the room, my first thought was, "Seriously! Doogie Howser?" He appeared to be roughly sixteen years old. In his 'infinite wisdom', he decided he would use a tens machine to numb the area around the incision. This machine is intended to send electrical impulses to the muscles, thereby helping to alleviate chronic pain. Since the incision was just below Shawn's heart, when this idiot applied the probes, his heart was sent into tachycardia. His body jolted off the bed like he had been hit with heart paddles – his eyes wide, searching, desperate for help. I held his hand and soaked his arm with my tears. I thought I was losing him.

I so wanted to punch 'Doogie Howser' in the head.

Just then, Pastor Dave from our church entered the room. He was a calming beacon of light, casting hope and assurance in our hearts. He was confused as to what was happening, but instantly recognized the fear in our eyes. His reassuring smile instilled serenity, amidst the increasing furor. His timing couldn't have been more perfect, as sheer panic was beginning to erupt. He had us join hands and we began to pray.

The nurses and doctors raced around the room, trying to get Shawn's heart rate under control. I looked at the monitor, which now revealed his heart had risen to two hundred and sixty beats per minute. I could see the panic on Shawn's face. He must have felt like a freight train was thundering through his chest. At this time, I'm sure my heart was racing right up there with his.

I closed my eyes tightly, trying to concentrate on the minister's voice. Soon a nurse ushered us out and asked that we wait in another room. The Pastor`s wife Maureen, was already in the waiting room, and this brought me much comfort. We all sat in a close circle with our hands joined. Dave and Maureen explained how they were able to be here with us, only by the grace of God.

I listened to their story:

They had arrived at the hospital in Ottawa, after travelling two hours from our hometown, only to discover that there was a restriction placed on Shawn's room. This was to limit the number of visitors, allowing only a few family and friends access. Pastor Dave told me how he had explained to the clerk that he was a close friend, there to provide spiritual guidance. Still he was refused entry. Dave lowered his head, realizing they had travelled this distance only to be turned away. But then, his eyes fell on a small piece of paper lying on the counter just in front of the admin clerk. He popped on his reading glasses and strained to see what was scrawled on the paper. He was almost certain it had Shawn's name with a room number beside it.

Pointing at the paper, Dave asked the clerk, "Is this him?"

The clerk replied, "Yes, I believe so. Isn't that strange! I never noticed that piece of paper laying there."

Dave asked, "Do you mind if I take it?"

Dumbfounded, the clerk replied, "By all means – take it." And she slid the piece of paper to Dave.

As he and Maureen walked away, Dave turned to see the clerk staring in bewilderment, still trying to comprehend what had just occurred.

After hearing their story, I felt a chill go through my body. I quickly dismissed it, thinking there must be some rational explanation. How fortunate we were that they had arrived when Shawn and I needed them most, not to mention how I needed them now. I explained to them how I had been walking along in a trance for days – and then it all came to the surface in blubbering sobs. I revealed my innermost, darkest fears.

I told them how I feared going back to the graveyard, with so many loved ones there: my cousin Julie, my dad, my uncle, and my aunt. They were all there in the same corner of the graveyard, and I couldn't bear to have Shawn there too. They listened, we prayed, and they comforted me.

Dave and Maureen were not strangers to us. They had been there since this nightmare began. Dave was retired, but he had covered for our regular pastor while he was on holidays. He was a dynamic speaker. For the first time in my life, I had felt that sermons were delivered directly through God's word. Let me clarify, I'm not overly religious, but Dave inspired me. He spoke of life lessons, real world issues, and related to everyone in the congregation through his stories and teachings. He spoke of being a good, honest person, and a contributing member of the community. He not only spoke of it, he lived it. Unfortunately, I had encountered many hypocrites in my lifetime who claimed to be devoted to the word of God, but who exemplified anything but Christian values.

Dave had taken Shawn under his wing, long before we learned about Shawn's illness, and he had become somewhat of a father figure. Shawn adored Dave, and I truly believe he came into our lives for a purpose.

In fact, I believe this with every fiber of my being. He was a messenger from God, there to carry Shawn through this ordeal by providing him with the inner peace he was searching for. This was so he would not die in fear.

Shawn's greatest fear was dying. That sounds strange coming from a man who served in the military, but Shawn was not certain there was a God or a heaven. He feared that he would no longer be on any plane, that he would turn to dust and all existence of his body and soul would cease to exist.

I was astounded when he told me this, not because I judged him, but because I wondered how anyone who lacked faith could survive losing a loved one. Faith is what carried me. Faith provided me with the certainty that I would be reunited with my loved ones, and had given me the strength in knowing my loved ones were safe and protected by God.

To be honest, I too have doubted the existence of God at certain times in my life, but my faith is renewed each time I experience miracles. And there have been many!

For instance,when Dave handed me the slip of paper he had found at the front desk. I immediately recognized my mother-in-law's handwriting. She had, for some reason, quickly written Shawn's name and room number on the piece of paper that morning, and then had forgotten it. I was mystified! How on earth had Dave found the note, which brought him and his wife to us, when we needed them most? The three of us joined hands in prayer, and this time Maureen spoke. She prayed that we would have strength. That we would walk with peace in our hearts, and that we would rejoice in God's ability to carry us. Her words were comforting and gave me the strength I needed to be there for my husband.

I went back to the hospital room after Shawn's heart rate had returned to normal levels. I held him in my arms and he started to cry.

He said, "You are going to think I am crazy, but I have to tell you something."

"Of course," I assured him, "you can tell me *anything*."

"Just after you left, when my heart was still racing, I felt warmth at my feet, as though someone was sitting against them. When I looked at the end of the bed, there sat the figure of a man. This man was surrounded with bright, yellow light, and although the light was blinding it didn't hurt my eyes. I asked him, 'Who are you? Are you God?' And he answered, 'No. I am the Son of God, and I am here to tell you to stop what you're doing. The cancer is gone from your body, but if you don't calm down, you will die.' I watched the monitor…watched as my heart rate dropped down to one hundred seventy-five beats per minute."

At first I didn't say a word. Could it be that Shawn had been visited by the Son of God? Of course, I tried to explain it away, thinking about all of the painkillers he had taken. Then, I looked into his eyes and knew he was telling the truth. I was certain it had happened, just as I was certain that many other people have experienced this when they are close to death.

Later that evening, I walked the two blocks back to the hotel. The hotel was sponsored by the Ronald McDonald House, which provided affordable accommodations for families of patients in long term care. Jarryd and Cole were back at our house with my sister, two brothers and sister-in-law who had all flown in from Alberta just a few days before. I was so grateful for their help. We had all agreed it would be unfair to ask a five and an eight year old boy to sit quietly in a hospital all day. I missed my boys terribly and felt torn, being away from them.

I remembered, I had packed my laptop on the off chance that I might get internet service, either at the hospital or in the hotel. At the very least, I could use it to do some writing and maybe send off an email later from home. I knew my family and friends were patiently waiting to hear how the surgery went and how Shawn was doing. I logged on to my Yahoo account, and surprisingly, I had internet service right away. I was able to write a long, heartfelt email to all of our friends and family.

My mother-in-law Denise entered the hotel room a few minutes later, insisting that I should get some sleep. I told her that I really needed to do this and that writing was cathartic and cleared my head. I read her the email:

> *Thursday, August 30, 2007*
>
> *Hi Everyone,*
>
> *Just a quick update on the surgery. Shawn was informed this morning that he is a very lucky man and that someone*

is definitely looking out for him – I know this in my heart! I believe my dad had a talk with God, telling him that Shawn is still needed here to look after his little girl and grandsons. We are not ready to let him go anywhere. He has done so much good on this earth and I believe he has been given a second chance at life. (I am convinced he is a cat, as this is not the first time he has brushed up with death).

The surgery went very well. Our biggest concern was that the cancer may have started to invade his liver. The surgeon told me that the liver is clear. That is when I started breathing again. But the stomach was completely overtaken with cancer, with a mass on top. They had to remove the entire stomach, the lower part of the esophagus, and all of the lymph nodes between the stomach and liver. The surgeon informed Shawn that he had never seen a stomach that infected, and that the lymph nodes were inflamed and rock hard. This is an indication that the lymph nodes were ready to invade the other organs, and this would have in turn traveled through the bloodstream, and he would have been given two months at best.

Shawn has a huge pain threshold. He never wanted to complain about all the pain he was experiencing this past year because he thought he had put me through enough with his job. You can imagine how awful I felt, knowing that he hadn't shared this with me.

Today has been a very difficult day, even more so than yesterday. Shawn's epidural did not take properly and he could feel all of the sutures and the opening of his two chest tubes. Shawn mentioned how his pain was a nine or ten out of ten most of the time. At one point, we were both in tears because he had just been through enough! Then our pastor came in and offered comfort through prayer, taking time with both of us individually to help us cope. It was amazing how he arrived, just when we needed him most. I am certain that faith and prayer were the forces driving everyone involved. I left the hospital at ten-forty-five this evening, and Shawn's new medication was taking effect. He remained positive through it all and was more worried about how he was putting everyone else out. The nurses were amazed at his strength, even though they could see his pain. The doctor came in before I left and gave us some great news: Shawn's white blood count is normal, so his body is fighting this enemy with a vengeance. We are certain that this thing will not get him! He has too much to do in this lifetime.

We love all of you and thank you for giving us strength. Shawn is overwhelmed with the love and prayers that have been sent and he knows he is a rich man. I believe riches are measured in the people you touch, and because of this, Shawn is one of the richest people I know.

Marie

I realized Denise had been crying throughout the letter. I stood up and embraced her, hoping to provide some comfort. Shawn was my husband, but I needed to remember, he was *her child*. Children are supposed to outlive their parents. This poor woman had lost her husband Ted just four years earlier, and now she feared she may lose her only son. I couldn't imagine what she must have been going through.

Denise bravely managed a smile and said, "That is simply beautiful! Would you be a dear – log on to my email account, and send the letter to my family as well? I'm sure they would love to hear how Shawn is doing."

I did exactly that, and as it was now after midnight, she suggested we get some much needed rest.

I jolted awake to the phone ringing at two a.m. It was the hospital asking that I return as soon as possible. They said Shawn was being transferred back to the intensive care unit – immediately! His heart had been racing for over two hours and they were trying desperately to get it under control. Frantically, I got dressed and ran the two blocks back to the hospital.

Luckily, Shawn had the heart of an ox, I think due to his regular physical activity, and he pulled through again.

The doctors told me later, that they were expecting to read him his last rites. They were calling him their 'Miracle Patient' and I believe he was.

Later that day, I went back to the hotel to get some sleep. First, I wanted to see if anyone had responded to the email I had sent. But when I opened the laptop, my eyes were immediately drawn to the x's covering the computer icons at the bottom of the screen. Had I been dreaming before? Did I really have a connection? Had I just imagined sending that letter?

Already prepared for what I knew I would hear, I called down to the front desk and tentatively asked the desk clerk, "Do you have internet service?"

She replied, "No, I'm very sorry. This is a budget hotel and we do not provide internet services."

I just about dropped the phone.

Again, I tried to explain it away, thinking I must have tapped into someone else's internet. But two days later, when Denise returned to my home, she checked her Google account. Every message I had sent from her account read 'Delivery Failure', and yet she had replies from every person we had sent the letter to. All of her contacts were saying they had received my email.

One coincidence, *fine*. Two coincidences, weird!

Three coincidences in twenty-four hours, I've got to put it out there – *miracle*.

The second miracle got me through the following year. After all, a visit from Jesus was not something to be scoffed at.

Chapter Five

Blindsided

Journal entry,

Tuesday, September 4, 2007

I always admired my mother for her strength, and somewhere along the way I hope I was blessed with some of that. Every time I have a weak moment or I need a rational, loving perspective, I have phoned my mom. She is a gift from God and she has always been there for me, to give me strength. When I question myself or something in my life, I trust that Mom will listen and give me some perspective. Even when she is being tough, she says the right things, which confirms how much she loves me. I only wish I could bottle some of her wisdom and assertion to give me the strength to get through times like this. She has a calmness about her. She never raises her voice, but still gets her point across effectively. People never take advantage of her, because she can read right through them. She stands her ground. Please give me some of that. I am the ultimate pleaser, never wanting to cause any waves. When I am with Shawn in the hospital, I put on a brave face, not wanting him to be afraid; meanwhile, I'm dying inside. I know how strong he is and how demeaning this disease can be. It can suck your energy and make you feel helpless. My Shawn has always conquered any challenge, but this one will be his biggest battle. The cancer is gone, but there is still a lot of fighting ahead. It's only when I see him feeling hopeless that I am afraid. With all that time to think and all those drugs on board, I can't imagine the internal battle. I imagine this is as frightening as any war. Any time your life is jeopardized, the feeling of helplessness is overwhelming. This all plays like a bad dream – I often can't accept that it's happening. Most days, I feel like a walking zombie. Sleep deprivation has taken a giant toll on us since this nightmare began. My mind cannot take information and process it effectively without sleep. Shawn has not been able to sleep more than one hour at a time and he often only gets fifteen to twenty minutes before he needs to push the button for pain control. It's Tuesday and he is finally in a private room where he can get two hours of sleep at a time. Finally, they found the proper antibiotic for the infection in his chest tube. He must feel like a guinea pig. The attachment of his small bowel to his esophagus was tested today and there is a moderate leak. They are giving it twenty-four hours to repair itself. The doc who performed the surgery was in today with his ICU team and he calls Shawn his 'miracle'. I am convinced he has a powerful team in heaven creating this miracle. We have been given a second chance.

A few months after Shawn's first surgery, I received a phone call from my mom. I could tell by the tone in her voice that she was upset. She said, "Your sister told me I had to phone you. She insisted that I couldn't keep it from you any longer, and that if I didn't tell you, she would."

"What is it, Mom? You're scaring me."

"Last summer, just before you moved to Ontario, I found a lump in my breast."

My tongue stuck to the roof of my mouth. I fell silent; retreating back into that familiar haze… I finally managed to spit out the word, "NO."

Mom's voice broke, "I didn't want to tell you, because I didn't want you to change all of your plans for me."

"Mom, that was over a year ago! Why didn't you tell me?"

"I didn't tell anyone," she said. "I told your sister only a month ago. I'd decided not to treat it, and I didn't want any of you talking me out of it."

"So you've been suffering in silence for over a year? Mom, I wouldn't have tried to talk you out of it, but I would have liked to have been there for you."

Mom continued, "I've watched people go through radiation and chemotherapy. I didn't want to go through that. I'm seventy-seven years old and I have had a good life."

"I understand you didn't want to go through the treatments. I completely understand that. What I don't understand, is you not telling anyone! You have always been there for the family. We have often leaned on you for support. We would have done the same for you. Shawn could have gotten out of his posting, and we could have stayed in Alberta. We could have been there to support you."

"You know me. I never wanted to be a burden to anyone."

Another truck hit me square in the face.

It all made sense now.

I remembered back to the day of Shawn's surgery, how I had called her then, and every chance I got. I needed my mother's help to get through this. She was still in Alberta, which made it difficult, and I remembered how she had apologized for not coming to Ontario. I knew she wasn't coming because she hated to travel. She didn't travel much at all anymore, telling me once after Dad died: "I lost my travel partner." But, I had also gotten the sense she was not feeling well. Come to think of it, she was uncharacteristically emotional the day we left Alberta and I remember thinking there was something more to her sadness

For the next six months, I travelled back to Alberta as much as possible. Mom was placed in a palliative care facility in January of 2008. Although, I myself could rarely be by her side, it gave me comfort to know my sister Suzanne was there every day, as well as my sister-in-law Kelly and cousin Joanne who spent many hours taking care of her.

Mom passed away June 2nd, 2008.

Chapter Six

Give Me Strength

The day after my mother passed away, our neighbours Judy and Vern, asked if they could treat Shawn and me to a nice dinner in town. Knowing we were flying home the next day, they hoped that the company would provide some small reprieve from our string of tragic events. Shawn wasn't feeling well, but came along anyway, because he knew it would mean a lot to them and to me. Judy and Vern's four children had offered to babysit Jarryd and Cole.

We had just ordered drinks when Judy received a call on her cell phone. I was sitting directly across from her and I witnessed the look of horror on her face. My first thought was, 'Someone else is dead! Then I began to pray, '*Dear God, please let my boys be safe.*'

Judy listened with sheer concern, and tears were now pooling in her eyes. She lowered the receiver and said, "Pepper bit Jarryd!"

It took a minute to register. Strangely, I felt relieved at first. After all, Pepper was a smaller dog – a French Brittany Spaniel. 'How much harm could he actually do?'

By the panic on Judy's face, I realized I didn't understand the seriousness of this. None of us were moving, frozen by the news.

Then Judy broke down, pleading, "Janet says it's real bad and she's not one to overreact. She called an ambulance. We have to get to the hospital right away! I'm so sorry! I'm so sorry!"

We immediately cancelled our order, threw some money on the table for our drinks, and Judy rushed us to the hospital.

The ambulance pulled in just as we did. Judy's van had barely come to a stop before I jumped out.

So many things were rushing through my head and I truly didn't know what to expect.

There was Jarryd. I could see him sitting on the bench seat in the back of the ambulance. He had a compression bandage covering his face, so I couldn't see the full extent of his injuries.

The paramedics lowered him into a wheelchair while I held his hand, and they rolled him inside. Then Jarryd lifted the bandage. My heart sank to my feet, but my face remained expressionless, for his sake. I managed to fake a comforting smile, while rubbing his hand and assuring him, "You're going to be fine, Jarryd. The doctors will take care of you." Meanwhile, I was screaming inside. I wanted to kill Pepper with my bare hands. Shawn was standing behind me, and I couldn't see his expression. My first thought, was that Shawn would be fine because he had witnessed many traumas in his military career. Surely he would maintain his composure.

Jarryd kept asking for a mirror, but we made every excuse not to give him one. We feared it would send him into hysterics. He was a tough kid, but this was shocking and ugly. He had been bitten clean through, from the tip of his lip, to his nose. He had this jagged, gaping bite on his cheek. All I could think was; how could they possibly repair this? *My beautiful little boy.*

Quickly, they got him into an examination room. The doctor completed his report, asking all sorts of questions about the incident. I was becoming impatient, thinking, shouldn't we get on with it? He told us Jarryd would need several sutures. Instantly, I started to think about how badly Jarryd would look if…and without hesitation asked,

"How confident are you in stitching him up?"

Caught off guard, the doctor stuttered a bit and then replied, "I have to be honest. This is not my specialty."

That was enough for me! Looking directly at Shawn, I stated, "We're driving to Ottawa."

He responded, "We are?"

I replied, "Yes we are! I know he's only a boy but he has to live with this face for the rest of his life. I want a plastic surgeon."

Shawn agreed with me. We got Jarryd and Cole into the car and settled in for the two hour drive to the Children's Hospital in Ottawa.

Jarryd was immediately assigned to a plastic surgeon and was given fifty sutures. We stayed with him, holding his hand while they froze the wounds and applied each stitch. Soon Shawn began to sob. He was holding Jarryd's hand tight, never wanting to let go, and he said, "My son needs me."

We both knew what he meant by this and I tried to be strong for all of us.

Shawn said, "I love you Jarryd."

"I love you too, Dad."

Then I lost it! I had to turn away. My life was falling down around me. How could this be happening?

A day later, we flew to Alberta to arrange for Mom's funeral. Jarryd had been given antibiotics to prevent infection, but overnight his face continued to swell. It had swollen so badly that he could barely move his head. We knew something was seriously wrong. So, while I was helping Suzanne make funeral arrangements, Shawn took Jarryd to see a doctor. Dr. Carter took one look at Jarryd and told Shawn to get him immediately to the Stollery Children's Hospital in Edmonton, as infection had set in.

Jarryd was given an MRI and underwent emergency surgery. He spent the entire week in the hospital. His wounds had to be reopened and drained. Every few hours the gauze was removed and repacked, over and over again, until all the infection was gone.

I sat by his bed thanking God he was all right.

Jarryd was released from the hospital just in time for his grandmother's funeral. The doctor told us it was a good thing we got him in when we did, because if the infection had spread any further, it would have entered into his bloodstream and then gone to his heart. I really don't know if I could have handled losing him too. That may have been the end of me.

Seriously, how much can a person take before they reach their breaking point?

A year later, it came out in counseling how the shock of this had traumatized both boys. Pepper had viciously latched on to Jarryd's face and would not let go. All of the kids were screaming hysterically, and there was blood *everywhere*. Judy and Vern's son Michael, pulled Pepper off Jarryd's face, but then Pepper turned on Cole – teeth bared and snarling, as if he'd gone mad. Terrified, Cole tried to push his body deeper in the couch, burying his face tight in his own arms, as he shook with fear. Michael reacted again, kicking Pepper hard, sending him flying into the nearest bedroom and locking the door. It all happened within a few seconds, but to Cole it seemed like an eternity.

Cole will never erase these images from his mind. Never to forget the ragged, bloody piece of Jarryd's skin hanging off Pepper's jowls as Pepper turned on him.

Jarryd underwent several treatments and two rounds of plastic surgery over the next two years. The surgeon at the Stollery Children's Hospital did an amazing job. To look at Jarryd today, you would never guess he had been mauled that severely.

Furthermore, I need to express how very proud I am of my son's bravery through this whole ordeal. I draw on Jarryd's strength every day. He perfectly exemplifies someone who is a survivor.

Chapter Seven

Letting Go

Shawn fought with everything he had. He endured five months of back to back chemotherapy and radiation. He actually went into remission for a few months, and we held strong in our faith that he would remain cancer free. We even started to make plans to return to Alberta, and Shawn was granted a transfer back to the military base in Edmonton.

The day before our flight back home to Alberta, Shawn was having difficulty breathing, and we discovered the cancer had returned. It was spreading throughout his lungs and abdominal cavity.

The doctors in Ottawa had made arrangements for Shawn to be admitted immediately to the University hospital in Edmonton. He spent only one month there before he was moved to a palliative care unit at the Grey Nuns Hospital. Still, Shawn never for a moment believed he would die. The doctors told us it was a miracle he had lived as long as he had, with such an aggressive case of gastric cancer.

Shawn's first surgery had been on August twenty-eighth, 2007, and he passed away August twelfth, 2008.

At first, I was very angry. After all, Jesus *himself* had come to tell us that all the cancer was gone. "What about that?" I cried, cursing the heavens.

But, I realized that the cancer had been gone, for a short time, while he was in remission. I believe God had come to give us hope and strength so that we could enjoy the time we had left together.

The gift we were given was one year. We were able to say everything we needed to say, and be a family for one last year.

I remembered the day I finally told him to let go. My dear friend Shelly had been sitting with him over several hours that week, and Shawn had confided in her that he would fight for as long as I needed him.

He had gone through enough pain.

There was nothing left of him – they had cut out half of his body and the machines were now keeping him alive. It would have been selfish of me to not give him permission to let go, although this was the hardest thing I have ever done in my life.

I caressed the back of his hand, feeling the warmth of his skin. Thinking, how many times had I grabbed his hand for strength, and how I needed to be strong for him now. I didn't know how my words would be received. Would he know that I wanted to let him go because I loved him with all my heart? Would he think he had been a burden to me all these months? I gathered all my strength…

"Shawn, you need to let go and be with God. The boys and I will be okay. You have endured enough pain. I need to let you go. I will join you when the time is right, but for now I will keep your spirit alive through our boys. I promise we will never forget you. You know how strong I am. I will take care of Jarryd and Cole, and protect them enough for both of us. I will always remind them of your love and your silly little sayings." I noticed a small smile form at the corner of his mouth as I said this.

I kissed his cheek – lingered there for a moment. "My dear sweet man, I will never stop loving you. Thank you for the best years of my life."

Sitting back on the chair, I placed my cheek on his furry arm, remembering the night we first met, trying to imagine my life without him. And I wept uncontrollably. My body heaved in pain, aching to have our life back. Our life that now played like a picture show flashing across a movie screen, segments filled with memories of days gone by.

Shawn returned the favour a week before he died, as he thanked me once again for being the girl of his dreams. While I sat holding his hand, he said, "Marie, after I am gone, you need to go on, and find love again."

I wouldn't hear of it! He could see my anger building. I began to sob, and yelled, "No, I don't want anyone else!"

He just talked right over me. "I need to give you permission, so you don't feel guilty. You have so much love to give. You have to *go on.*" He pleaded.

To this day, I still can't imagine how difficult this was for him. It only proves how well he knew me, how deeply he loved me, and how unselfish he was.

My dear, sweet husband – *I will always love you.*

Chapter Eight

Crossing Over

"The body may falter but the spirit shines on–
lighting the way to strength, courage and hope,
just as the sunshine lights a new day."

–Anonymous

The drip of the machines and the sleep-induced state left him light as a cloud. He could hear faint voices becoming more distant…

His body was below him now as he was lifted to another dimension, another world - this one filled with fields of violet blossoms as far as the eye could see. He looked to his side and saw that he was holding someone's hand. She was *beautiful*. She had a soft, calming smile that lifted just at the corners of her mouth. Her lips, stretched in a thin line, portrayed an air of confidence and utter serenity. He felt he had known her his entire life…only he had never set eyes on her before. Now surrendering, he allowed her to guide him through this magical world, without questioning.

Deep down, he knew he had left his mortal world and life behind for greater things – then suddenly, he remembered his wife and sons. He felt a loss that bit at the back of his throat and radiated through his stomach and then his loins.

Would he ever see them again, hold them in his arms, and feel that safe, penetrating love?

Would he see his boys grow, love, hurt, and experience life?

Then, he took a moment to look over his body. The body that was filled with disease. The body that had transformed into something he didn't know. It had withered, shrunk, and aged beyond recognition. His body, which he had pushed to the point of breaking so many times in the military and in the weight room, had *failed him*.

But now as he looked, he realized his body had regained its strength and youth. He raised his face to the sun and let the warmth quench his skin with a penetrating renewal. He *rejoiced* in the moment.

He said, "*There is a God*." And he laughed with relief!

He had asked that question so many times, and now the answer was revealed. He thought of how he had desperately wanted to believe there was a God, and how he had longed for unshakable faith, remembering how even in his darkest hours, he had questioned his eternal existence.

Now remembering his beautiful wife, he desperately wanted to share his joy with her. But a twinge of anger interrupted his bliss – was this the trade off? What a cruel joke. He had his body back, but what good was it to him now, when he no longer shared the same earthly plane as his wife and children?

What were they doing now? How were they going to get through all of the details: the funeral, the pain, the road ahead?

He realized that the girl was still holding his hand, and finally he asked, "Who are you?"

She responded, "I am your guardian, and I am here to lead you through the afterlife."

With bitter sarcasm, he laughed again. This must be *a dream*. Then he remembered the conversation he had with Marie about the afterlife. He had been convinced that when he died, he would simply be dust. This was what he feared most about dying:

To be nothing.

To have gone through life, to end up worm meal.

To have absolutely *no brain activity.*

But, Marie said she was certain that there was a heaven and he would be reacquainted with the loved ones who had passed before him. He remembered how she had talked him through it and he had tried to believe her, but still couldn't rid himself of the terrible uncertainty, his fear that was buried deep within.

Now he wanted desperately to share this with Marie, to tell her she was right!

He wanted to share everything with her, but he knew she was gone. He felt his heart weigh heavy in his chest, with the burden of everything he had gone through. It all came swelling to the surface in tremendous sobs. The sobs began in his stomach and burned. He wondered if the heavens felt every ounce of his pain. He cried for his kids, his wife, his mother, and all of the wretched surgeries and treatments his body had experienced. Most of all, he cried for himself.

The unfairness ripped through him like a thousand painful lashes.

He looked to his right and there she was – this angel. Tears also streaked her cheeks, and he saw that she felt his pain as deeply as he did. She could read his thoughts and feel his anguish as though they were her own.

He felt an overwhelming blanket of protection, as the realization set in – he would never be alone.

Chapter Nine

A Safe Haven

After Shawn died, I wanted to curl up in a ball and sleep forever, but I had two young boys and Lexi to care for, so this was not an option. I was fortunate that I didn't have to return to work immediately.

Besides, none of us were sleeping particularly well, and if we did sleep, dreams revealed our new reality, and we woke up cranky, depressed and filled with fatigue. Most mornings consisted of outbursts and meltdowns, and this drained our energy even before we walked out the door. I can't begin to describe how grateful I was that I didn't have to rush to a job as well.

While it probably would have been easier to stay in bed all day and not deal with reality, I felt it was important for myself and my boys to keep things as normal as possible. They got to school every day, even if that meant waiting in the truck until they were ready to go inside, showing up an hour late, or crying on the sleeve of the school counselor until they were able to go to class. Whatever it took, we had to continue.

Lexi helped me establish a routine. At the sound of the alarm clock, Lexi would take her cue and jump up on the boys' beds to get her fill of cuddles and licks. The boys would be covered with slobber, but it didn't matter, because to hear them giggle was the best part of my day.

Once the boys were ready for school, we would jump in the SUV, and if the weather permitted, we would roll down the window and Lexi would stick her big head out. She must have been quite the sight for the other commuters. The rushing air would get trapped under her lips, making the sound of a flag flapping in the wind. Meanwhile, her ears would do a separate dance. She would close her eyes, maybe in satisfaction, or maybe just so the drool wouldn't fly into her eyes. She was completely content, and appeared to have a smile on her face.

After the kids were settled at school, I would drive to Timmy's to get my morning coffee. Lexi would still have her head stuck out the window, because she knew if she showered them with cuteness, the attendant at the drive-thru would typically offer her a plain Timbit. Oh yeah, she knew how to work the system! She would take the Timbit ever so gently into her mouth, and devour it in one gulp.

Our next stop would be the big open field just behind our subdivision. The field looked more like a gravel pit, as it had become the official dumping ground for the dirt and sand left over from the new houses being built. I was informed that it was to be leveled at a later date for more residential development, but for now all that existed was an open expanse. At the very center of the field lay a massive crater-like hole, where my boys were convinced a UFO had once landed. I laughed at their imaginative stories and could see why they believed this. It certainly did appear to be something straight out of *Close Encounters of the Third Kind*.

I would take Lexi off her leash and she would break into a run, tearing up and down the dirt hills. Then she would sniff around the field and dig at new holes she found. This was my time to sit with my coffee and calm down from the morning insanity. I would linger in my thoughts and eventually Lexi would wander over, lean her full weight into my side, and kiss my face as if to assure me I was not alone. There we would rest, my arm draped around her. Sometimes the tears would come, but more often I felt at peace. Lexi and I would tilt our heads to the sky and bask in the warmth of the sun penetrating deeply, as though Shawn's arms embraced us.

Now that I think back, this place became a sort of safe haven for the boys too. They spent a lot of time there. They would use a crazy carpet or a sled to slide down the sides of the crevices. It didn't matter, summer or winter, snow or dirt, as long as they could slide down those hills. Funny, it wasn't the prettiest place in the world, but somehow we were all drawn to it. Free of all the chaos, no one could disturb us there.

There is something to be said about the starkness of barren land. We were comforted, perhaps because our lives felt empty since Shawn had passed. The huge crater symbolized the hollowness in our hearts. In some strange way, the field brought us closer to Shawn and to God.

Chapter Ten

Shawn

He began to tour this place called heaven. Never in his wildest dreams had he imagined it this way. Everything was unspoiled, like going back to the beginning of time with pure, crystal clear water and lush green vegetation. The trees were majestic – standing proud and tall, undisturbed by man. Everything in this world was amazingly bold. It reminded him of getting a new pair of glasses, with the pristine lenses sharpening the clarity of everything around you.

He finally thought to ask the girl her name. She answered, "My name is Raya."

She spoke with a gentleness that calmed the soul and provided him with an inner peace. She gave him hope that he would heal in every way. His bruised and battered heart would mend and grow whole again. His body, ravaged by the numerous surgeries, would be repaired and intact.

He thought of how difficult it had been to wake up after each surgery, in a semi-conscious, highly medicated state, and learn that yet another part of his body had been removed. This had been incredibly demeaning. He had been at the mercy of the doctors, and they had been at the mercy of medical research. It had been a tragic comedy of hits and misses. He had become a human guinea pig. Meanwhile, what quality of life had he suffered? They had taken his entire stomach, twenty-seven lymph nodes, the lower half of his esophagus, and had given him a bag to poop in. He had become a feeble, aged, angry, and defeated forty-two year old, and he had endured a slow, painful death – one surgery at a time.

But now he was whole again! He wanted to scream to the heavens and run through the endless fields before him, yell at the top of his lungs until his throat bled. At the same time, he wanted to punch something with all of his strength, to release the anger that ripped through him. He remembered once being asked if it were possible to feel two emotions at the very same time. His answer now was "Hell yes!" He had felt unbearably tormented, having no control of his life. He remembered lying in that hospital bed day after day – just taking it. How could he have just accepted his dignity being stripped away? He had pent up his emotions for what seemed an eternity, and now it needed to come out, to explode!

But there were also *regrets*. If only he had more time. He would have spent every spare minute with his boys and he would have made more of an effort to indulge in their moments. He had let countless opportunities pass without bathing in their beauty. He had spent far too much time obsessing about work, and he had rarely dropped everything to just play and engage with his family. Why? Why did he not anticipate how short life could be? Now that it was too late, he realized that whether a person lives eighty years or forty-two years, if they don't take time to hold their loved ones and really listen to them, they are cheating themselves out of the gift of life.

Yes, if he could do it all again, he would drop everything just to look into the eyes of his wife and sons and bask in the glory that lay there. He thought if he could pass any message back to Earth, it would be to live in each moment and soak up every delectable morsel that life offers. Not run through life, but instead take a stroll, and live every day as though it were your last.

The tears welled and tore through his body in gut wrenching sobs. As he cried, the sky above him opened with a loud crash, and rain pelted down, drenching his body.

He cried so hard he thought he could never cry again…but he was wrong. He would, and the next time his tears would not be for his own sad tale.

He looked at Raya, who gently reached out to hold his hand. Then she placed her other hand on his shoulder. And, as she did this, it felt familiar – his mind took him back to a time when he and Marie had just started dating.

The white Pontiac Grand Am was but a week old. He was burning the candle at both ends – working eight hour days in the Military, and working for another company doing house inspections at night. It was September, and Marie had just started the school year. She too was exhausted, busy preparing lessons and year plans for her students. But still, she had asked to come along, worried that he might fall asleep.

They stopped at Timmy's and loaded up on large coffees for the trip out of town. Marie still couldn't keep her eyes open, so she tilted the seat all the way back, begging for ten minutes of sleep.

The next thing he heard was Marie screaming at the top of her lungs. He jolted awake to see that they were now in the middle of the double highway and the Grand Am, trying its best to cut through the tall grass, was spitting the terrain up into large clumps over the hood.

Now fully awake, he recalled how he had put the car on cruise control, and realized he must have drifted off.

Marie was still screaming, but somehow he remained completely calm. With one hand on her knee and the other hand still controlling the steering wheel, he attempted to calm her down, saying, "It's okay Marie. It's okay!"

He remembered a hand on his shoulder, guiding him and keeping him calm.

He knew exactly what to do and Marie was amazed at his composure. He thought Marie would surely put her foot through the floorboards, but he himself never once touched the brakes. Instead, he slowly maneuvered the car through the ditch and back on the road, meanwhile shoulder checking for oncoming traffic.

When he got back on the road, Marie was furious! She jumped out of the car, swearing a blue streak and yelling at his stupidity. She swore he would NEVER, EVER drive her car again!

He really couldn't blame her, and now as he thought back, it was comical how it all played out. They laughed about it later, saying how they must have looked like something out of *The Dukes of Hazard* to the other commuters on the highway.

He did as he was told and didn't dare touch her car for over a week. The amazing thing was that there was no damage to the car at all, just some grass jammed into the front undercarriage and bumper. They had been going one hundred and twenty kilometers per hour on cruise control. The highway was twinned and there was a ditch between the four lanes, and that was where they had found themselves when they woke up.

The next time they drove that highway, they took notice that there were very few straight stretches in that ditch without some kind of obstacle – there were many cross roads, several culverts, uneven ground, and large debris. It was miraculous that they had survived, and even more amazing that neither of them had been seriously injured. Shawn recalled how his composure had been uncanny, and remembered how Marie had thanked him a few days later, after she finally calmed down.

It was then that he told her how he had felt a presence there with him, guiding him, keeping him completely calm. He remembered telling Marie he believed it was his guardian angel. And now, he was certain of it, for the hand he had felt on his shoulder that day was the very same hand he felt now. Tears welled in his eyes as he gratefully acknowledged Raya, "That was you."

Raya simply nodded and smiled.

"Thank you Raya. Thank you *with all my heart*."

Chapter Eleven

Meeting Loved Ones

Raya guided him along a path through a field overflowing with radiant purple flowers – *Marie's favourite colour* he thought, and suddenly, he understood why she loved it. Purple is calming and vibrant, magical and warming. It wraps you in a blanket of joy and gives you faith and empowerment.

The path led to a river, and on the river was a canoe. There were two people paddling the canoe and playfully arguing. The woman was matter-of-fact and the man was hamming it up. He was teasing her, and although she looked annoyed, Shawn could tell she loved this playful banter. They were bickering about which direction they should go. He insisted that the easiest way to go around the mountain was west, while she insisted that they go east. This went on for some time, and he finally gave into her. It turned out she was right, because the flow of the river would provide the least resistance if they did, in fact, go east. She didn't say, '*I told you so.*' But she might as well have. She gloated a bit and he retorted with some wise crack about her being 'an old bird.'

'Old bird'. Where had he heard that before?

Shawn stopped in his tracks and looked closer. "Is that you, Vivian?"

She looked back and almost dropped her paddle. Her face lit up, and she sat paralyzed for a moment. Then her voice pierced the air in a high pitched scream of excitement as she shrieked, "Shawn? Is that you? Oh my God, Romeo, it's Shawn!"

"Shawn who?"

Getting annoyed with him, she replied, "Marie's husband, that's who!"

"Marie, our daughter?"

"Yes, of course our daughter! Keep up."

They paddled as fast as they could to reach him. He ran into the water, waving his arms. His chest felt heavy, as though a horse was standing on it. He could barely catch his breath. He was ecstatic to see her! Marie had told him he would be reunited with his loved ones, but he hadn't believed her.

He remembered how Vivian had passed away two months before him, and how dearly Marie loved her. He thought of Vivian's dry sense of humour, how she sometimes appeared to be almost cold on the outside, but she really had a heart of gold. She always spoke her mind, and people adored that about her. She was not mean spirited, but more like an *eye opener.* With Vivian, it was 'what you see is what you get.' People appreciated her consistent nature. She was always to the point, and had this genuine wisdom. She listened more than she talked and you always knew who you were talking to. She didn't seem to be affected by pesky hormones and mood swings like other women. She was constant and nurturing, in a no-nonsense way.

Shawn adored her and couldn't wait to give her a big, old, mushy hug. Vivian hated mushiness, but Shawn loved to tease her.

Vivian jumped out of the boat, well before it reached the shore, and ran through the water towards Shawn. She threw her arms around his neck and gave him a huge bear-hug. They laughed like children and fell in the water, still embracing.

Romeo calmly paddled to the shore, pulling the boat up on the sand before he walked over. He had this gorgeous smile, so genuine and welcoming. He made every person feel like they were the only important one in the universe. Shawn finally understood what Marie had meant when she said her dad could light up a room and everyone in it. Marie had said, he didn't have a single enemy that she knew of, and if there was anyone who didn't like her dad, it was probably because they were jealous. For he was loving in nature and pure of heart.

Shawn noticed Romeo's dimple right away, the same dimple his son Cole had. Ironically, he and Marie had given Cole the middle name Romeo. It was as if they knew! Like his grandfather, Cole was a flirt and a tease, he was slow as molasses in the spring, and he loved to hear himself talk and sing. Shawn loved Romeo instantly, and with all the stories Marie had shared, he felt he already knew him.

Romeo had the handshake of a man who was confident about himself. Shawn looked straight into those hazel eyes and said, "I never thought I would ever have the pleasure of knowing you. Marie told me everything about you. My God, she loves you!" Shawn blushed a little, because the words had all came rushing out of his mouth without thinking.

With a smile, Romeo replied, "The pleasure is all mine, son. To finally meet the man who gave my daughter two beautiful children, the man who loves her the way you do. Thank you for taking care of my little girl in my absence."

Shawn bombarded them with questions. "When did you and Romeo meet up again? How long did it take you to cross over? You both look just great!"

Vivian raised her hands in front of her like a police officer halting traffic, "Slow down young fellow; you are going to give yourself a stroke!" then began to laugh at the absurdity of it all.

Shawn laughed with her and said to Romeo, "God, I missed this woman!"

Romeo chuckled, "Good, feel free to take her off my hands for a while."

Vivian completely ignored Romeo's comment and addressed Shawn. "Last time I saw you, I told you to keep your pecker up! It is obvious you didn't listen to me. What are you doing here with us old folks? You were supposed to have a long life, and watch those boys…" She stopped mid-sentence, realizing she had gone too far.

A mixture of emotions rushed through Shawn. He was half-smirking at her wit, but felt a sting when he thought of his young sons Jarryd and Cole, who would go through life without him.

Romeo gave her a hard nudge on the shoulder, followed by a sharp look.

She attempted to correct herself by saying, "I mean, I thought you were on the mend. We all thought you'd beat it. What happened?"

Shawn explained how the cancer had gone into remission for a short time but then, it had spread. Romeo and Vivian listened with concern and sadness.

"Marie is one tough cookie," Shawn assured them.

"I know, and I'm sure she and the kids will be fine," Romeo added.

"She is strong, but I still think she needs to be tougher with those kids," Vivian replied.

Romeo gave her another nudge in the shoulder and shot her another look.

"Well, it's true. I always thought she was too soft with them."

Shawn exchanged a smile with Romeo, just to assure him it was okay. He felt Vivian could say anything right now, and he would still feel happy. For he was here with people he loved, in this amazing place. Most of all, he was no longer alone, and was now blessed with the opportunity to know his father-in-law. He suddenly remembered Raya. 'How could I be so rude?' he thought. But when he turned, she was gone.

Chapter Twelve

Marie

I awoke from a dream…

The tears came in buckets, washing away all of the pent up sadness. I vividly recalled his face, as though he were standing right in front of me. Sobbing into my pillow, I ached to hold him again.

This was the first time I had dreamt of Shawn since he died, at least to my recollection. I replayed the dream in my mind – how he had stood barely a foot away, with his back to me. At first, it wasn't clear who he was, but then he turned, and I gasped. He looked just as I had remembered! His body had transformed back into the man he was before the illness had robbed him.

I remembered, wanting to reach out in my sleep to touch that adorable, toothy grin, watching his mouth move, seeing him smile.

The tears came again…they came hard, wracking my body.

Emptiness remained in my stomach.

I thought of how he had fought with everything he had, enduring five months of back to back chemotherapy and radiation, and for what?

I grasped the pillow with both hands and squeezed with all my strength, clenching my teeth in hatred of this miserable, debilitating disease that steals our loved ones away and leaves us helpless.

But then, my anger began to soften, and I spoke the words aloud, "*We were given an extra year with him.*"

Then it came to me. He had visited so that I would know he was happy.

He had spoken a name: "Raya." What did it mean?

I quickly ran downstairs to my computer and searched the name's meaning. Raya: Hebrew (Israeli origin); gender – female; meaning wise guardian; also friend or companion.

Chapter Thirteen

Faith

While I read through my emails the next morning, I came across a saved folder. When I opened the folder, I saw it contained a message from our neighbour Vern, in Ontario. He and Shawn had become close friends, and each would often venture out into the yard if one of them was in the proverbial 'doghouse', or if they needed to get away from the chaos. Yes, they would casually sneak away and meet to contemplate life. Funny, it always reminded me of the sitcom *Home Improvement* with Tim Taylor and his neighbour Wilson.

I was puzzled. Vern must have written this letter while I was making preparations for the funeral, but for the life of me I didn't remember reading it, much less saving it to a folder.

August 15, 2008

Dear Marie,

I would like to gather my thoughts about Shawn.

My first memory is the day you moved in. I could tell from the firm handshake and the bright, sparkling, blue eyes that looked directly at mine that here was a good guy and we would be friends. Every one of the many short encounters we had over the next few days made me like him more and more. He did become a good friend and I don't make many friends. I am friendly with a lot of people, but few of them I truly consider friends.

Do only the good die young? Definitely, in this case. As you said, he must have had little left to accomplish in this life. A good God could only allow this to happen because somehow in the bigger scheme of things, Shawn had gotten done what needed to get done.

From my perspective, a man with very similar goals and aspirations for life and the future of my family, his passing was far too soon, and I have been asking why now, when there is still so much that needs to be done?

But Shawn consoled me when I told him that I felt robbed of our friendship, and yet he said we had to trust that there was a reason. We had talked earlier of faith and in the end this has been a challenge, but Shawn chose to trust God without making sense of what seemed left undone in his life, and I feel compelled to follow his lead. That to me is truly an inspiration and example, because really what is faith if not that?

I know he wanted only to be able to see his sons Jarryd and Cole, and his daughters Amber and Jasmine, to grow up healthy and happy. Every good father would feel the same. I know he overcame many obstacles in life and I believe his children will be able to do the same, despite such an awful blow, with the help of family and through the memory of their dad.

He didn't want to leave them now, but if there is one thing I think he would want them to have from him, it would be that spirit of not feeling sorry for yourself. Just get it done and always do the right thing by others.

He knew he wasn't perfect, as none of us are, but I told him that even though I had been on this earth longer than he, I looked up to him and admired him. I said this to him because he was able to use what he had been given (not dwelling on what he never had or on what had been taken from him) to improve his life and the lives of the ones he loved. That will be my lasting memory of Shawn.

We won't be able to be with you to celebrate Shawn's life but we continue to ask God to bless everyone in this time of sorrow.

Love Vern

I responded,

December 20, 2008

Dear Vern,

I found your letter saved in a folder, and for the life of me don't remember receiving it or saving it. As it turns out, I read it just now, at a time when I most needed it, and it touched me deeply. You are truly a great man; don't ever forget that. That is why you and Shawn shared a bond.

Christmas is just a few days away and we have prepared a celebration for Shawn. His stocking went up at the request of the boys. I really didn't know what to do, but they said we needed to put it up. Yesterday, Cole and I bought four candles and four beautiful ornaments: one for each of us, and Nana too. We plan to light a candle on Christmas and each place an ornament on the tree. Instead of trying not to cry or think of him, we plan to share stories and pictures of his time with us. It was much too short, but we have to feel blessed for the time we had.

There is definitely emptiness, but I feel that he is here guiding us. When I look at Lexi, I realize that this was Shawn's plan – to make sure we were not alone and always protected. Lexi really is a sweetheart and she has been a companion for me when I am here at home. She also gets me out for walks.

I was given a book by Shawn's cousin Lisa when I was in Florida. The book is called The Shack by William P. Young, and it changed my life. When I started reading the book, I was in the anger phase of my grieving, and was cursing everyone and everything. I couldn't believe that a loving God could make the boys and I endure so much in one year.

I could identify with the main character in a way that is unexplainable, even to me. I was questioning God and what seemed to be his wrath. I stopped going to church and didn't speak about God for months. I started to believe that Shawn was right, that we were dust when we died, and this threw me into utter despair. I was angry and felt pain beyond what anyone could imagine. I didn't know what my purpose was, so I simply went through the motions in life, without any joy. I felt terrible for Cole and Jarryd, because they had lost their grandmother, their father, and now they were losing their mom, but in a different way. They were acting up terribly, and I realize now it was because I had lost that attachment with them. They just wanted Mom back!

I couldn't put the book down; it had such a grip on me. I remember the boys were lying in bed with me, watching a movie on TV, as I continued to read and read. Finally, Jarryd asked me why I was so interested in the book, and what came out of my mouth was miraculous.

I told my children how, for the first time in my life, I had learned what God was about. I suddenly understood the meaning of suffering and identifying with God instead of turning to him only when times were tough. God didn't wish this upon us, but instead grieved with us, and felt the intensity of pain he felt when humanity had turned on his son. I realized that God would be there when I felt alone and that the Holy Spirit would be there to help me build my garden (this will make much more sense when you read the book).

And when I finished the book, I realized that most of my pain came from guilt. I felt guilty that I didn't know Shawn had cancer, and that I thought nothing could ever happen to him. I didn't take it seriously when he complained about his stomach. I just thought he wanted attention (like any man – when he is sick), so I would say something cute or sarcastic. I could not forgive myself for that!

But then, I realized that this was bigger than me, and as Shawn would say, "There is no axis up my butt." I can't control everything! The only one who can is God, and it was not even God who made this happen; it was a man-made disease and humanity wants to advance at any cost. God feels the pain from our mistakes, but will never leave us. Like loving parents, God allows us to make mistakes and feels our pain as deeply as we do, but in the end, we either learn from our mistakes, or we continue to make them. As I said, I couldn't control this; it was much bigger than me.

"This is my long winded sermon of the day." My point is you need to read this book.

Have a wonderful Christmas.

Love Marie

Chapter Fourteen

Walking Zombie Woman

I was out driving in the truck when the music on the radio was interrupted by a phone call. On the other line, was a military police officer from the Edmonton Garrison. "Oh no," I thought, "was I speeding? Oh great! Another photo radar ticket to add to the collection." I braced myself to hear what I had done.

"Ma'am, I don't really know how to say this. There have been a few items dropped off at the detachment, and I have been trying my best to track down who they belong to."

I listened carefully, intrigued now.

"The items are: two miniature urns, a beret, some military medals and some cuff links. They were discovered by a gentleman who works at the waste management station in town. He knew they must be important, so he dropped them off here at the base, hoping to find the owners. Ma'am, I did the research and discovered that one of the urns contains the ashes of a Mr. Edward Carr and the other contains the ashes of a Mr. Shawn Reed. I just got off the phone with a Mrs. Denise Reed-Carr in New Brunswick. She says she is your mother-in-law, and confirmed that Mr. Edward Carr (Ted) was her late husband. She asked me to contact you, saying that the other urn contained the ashes of your late husband (her son). Is this correct, Ma'am?"

I was very confused, my mind now swarming for answers. I sat silently for a few moments, and then remembered the bag Denise had handed me before she went back to New Brunswick. The bag which contained these very items. "Oh shit!" I thought.

"Ma'am, Mrs. Carr said I should call you to pick up these items. Would you be willing to do that?"

"Yes, I'll pick them up," I said, my heart now in my feet. "I can come by tomorrow. I would come today but my son has piano lessons."

"Thank you Ma'am. I will leave them here at the police detachment for you to pick up, labeled with your name."

I started to wrack my brain, trying to remember how on earth these things had ended up in the garbage. Suddenly, it all came back, how my mother-in-law had placed the bag in my hands saying, "Marie, I am entrusting you with my Ted and my Shawn. I don't want to risk taking them with me on the airplane, in case they are lost. Please take good care of them."

I felt like a complete fool! I must have been in a daze, as I vaguely remember putting the bag on the top shelf in the laundry room closet. My mind struggled for answers: Had it fallen off the shelf onto the floor? Did someone pick it up and put it in the garbage? Maybe my cleaning service? It was just a plastic grocery bag with a bunch of other grocery bags inside, individually wrapping each of the items. But it definitely must have had some weight to it. Who? What? Why?

My heart was racing and I could feel my face heating up with embarrassment. What had I done? Denise was going to kill me!

I cried out, "Oh my God, oh my God – I am so dead!"

I swear, even Lexi in the back seat had that "Uh Oh" look on her face.

I knew that lately my life had become a comedy of errors, but this took the cake. "Okay folks, time to round up the sacrificial gods and chuck me off the cliff. Please put me out of my misery before Denise gets to me."

But I sucked it up, and immediately called her, pleading for forgiveness…and being the kind, forgiving soul she is, my mother-in-law instantly forgave me.

I have included two emails Denise received. The first email is from Fabian, the employee who originally found the items at the recycling station, and the other email is from his brother William:

August 14, 2010

Do you know an Edward Ted Carr?

I have some very sentimental items of his. If you don't that is okay, but the name I am looking for is the same as yours. I am using my brother's Facebook account to send this...which is why I am leaving my email address.

Sincerely,

Fabian

Denise completely disregarded this first email, thinking it was suspicious. After all, why would a total stranger have sentimental items belonging to her late husband? Fortunately, Denise had taped a small label to Ted's urn where she had written: his name, the date he had passed, and the name of the funeral home in New Brunswick. This is how the military had been able to track her down.

She saved Fabian's email and two months later received this email from Fabian's brother:

October 10, 2010

Denise

It was my brother Fabian and his crew who found them at a recycle company they work at. My bro has no FB so he used mine to try to find you or anyone else in the Carr family. They went through the shredder and for some reason, they were not destroyed. It was like they had a mission that continued on after death, and so the journey began for my brother and his crew - the journey to find home. Now we found you, this journey and mystery shall have a positive ending - to make this speech short...

Thank you

William

My heart overflows with gratitude for this loving gesture. This from two brothers who were complete strangers to us, but who made it their mission to find us, and then later took the time to write this heartfelt sentiment to our family.

Once again, we were blessed with a miracle.

Chapter Fifteen

One Step at a Time

Everything in the new house reminded me of Shawn, especially all of the tools in the garage, which had been packed by a moving company in Ontario, and then moved to Alberta, only to be unpacked again. I hadn't the foggiest clue how to use most of the tools and now saw them as a continuous reminder of the lack of control I had over my life. I thought for a moment it would be easier to just have a yard sale – but then I remembered a promise I had made to Shawn one day in our garage back in Ontario.

We were getting the boat ready for winter and storing everything in big plastic bins with lids. Vern had come across the street to give us a hand. Just as we were busily sorting and packing, Shawn stopped in his tracks, stood in the middle of the garage, and looked around. It was as if it was the first time he had ever taken stock of this inventory. His favourite saying was, "The right tool for the right job," and I am certain he had acquired every tool for every job.

Looking back, I believe it struck him at that moment – knowing he may have to decide what would be done with all of the tools he had collected over the years. His shoulders slumped in defeat and he looked like a lost soul. The pit of my stomach twisted as his pain became mine.

In all of this, our lives had morphed into something foreign. We no longer understood our purpose. It was frightening! Our fate was in the hands of someone or something else. As I looked at my husband, I noticed that his vibrant blue eyes were now dull remnants of his once beautiful life. The sparkle was gone, and an old person now occupied his body.

He said, "I want you to keep all of these tools for my boys. Marie, please promise me you won't sell them."

I had been running on adrenaline all these months, and had convinced myself that he would be among that thirty percent who survive this horrible disease. But when I really looked at him, I froze in my tracks. He stood helpless, like an innocent child, surrendering to this demon disease. For the first time in months, I fully understood what was happening here. He was going to die! Like a lightning bolt, it hit us, and then the tears came with a vengeance.

Poor Vern walked in at that moment to ask a question, but quickly averted his eyes and walked back out. We were holding each other with every thread of dignity we had left. Stripped of our hopes and dreams, we were forced to accept a new path of existence.

My walks with Lexi continued. We would often go to the field or dog park, and at least twice a week we would visit the graveyard.

Lexi loves to rip around the graveyard and track through the trees to the wheat fields beyond. This place always fills my heart with endearing sentiment, for the fields in which she frolicks are the same fields my father farmed while I was growing up. The serene little sanctuary consists of a church, a hall, and about a dozen farmhouses. It had been a farming community for more than a century, with each plot of land handed down by birthright, usually to the oldest son.

My father's grandfather built our house – a large, red-bricked two-story home, one of three in our community, and where my oldest brother still lives today. People often compare our little hamlet of Lamoureux to small communities commonly found in Quebec – with its old styled buildings and century aged trees, lining a narrow country road that winds along the North Saskatchewan River.

The cemetery is located just behind the family farm, behind the church, and down a dusty road that cuts through the wheat fields.

My dad's grave is just on the edge of the trees of his property. The family did this purposely; that way, he could still look out onto the crops and oversee the family farm. He had tried to retire several times, but farming was in his blood and he never did give it up. After his nephew took over, he still had his hands in it, usually helping to remove the final yield. He complained about farming until the day he died, but always with a tone of endearment.

When Mom and Shawn passed away, they joined Dad in that quaint little corner of the cemetery. Mom's ashes were to be interred on August twenty-first, on her seventy-eighth birthday. At the time, the family was unaware that Shawn's funeral would be just two days prior.

I remember arriving that day with Denise, Jarryd, and Cole, placing a beautiful wreath Shawn's grave, then taking just five steps to where Mom's ashes were to be laid.

Many times I walk among their graves: my mother, father, husband, uncle, aunt, and cousin. I speculate on the meaning of life and how all these people I love have departed this earth. But, surreal as it is, being there provides some peace within me – just knowing they are all together.

Each time I stand beside Shawn's grave, I read the inscription and feel comfort.

"One equal temper of heroic hearts.
Made weak by time and fate, but strong in will.
To strive, to seek, to find and not to yield. By Tennyson

These words were etched in my memory from the first moment I read them. They are lines from the poem "Ulysses" by Lord Alfred Tennyson. I first read the passage in my university days, well before Shawn and I met. These three lines are only a small part of the passage, but I would like to briefly explain: Ulysses and his fellow warriors are trying to return home after The Battle of Troy. They face torrential rainstorms and deadly tides created by the god Poseidon, who tries to take them down. Meanwhile, at home, his wife Penelope fears that he is dead, but she never gives up hope.

The section of the poem leading up to the last three lines reads:

Tis not too late to seek a newer world.
Push off, and sitting well in order smite.
The sounding furrows; for my purpose holds
To sail beyond the sunset, and the baths
Of all the western stars, until I die.
It may be that the gulfs will wash us down;
It may be we shall touch the Happy Isles,
And see the great Achilles, whom we knew.
Though much is taken, much abides; and though
We are not now that strength which in old days
Moved earth and heaven, that which we are, we are;
One equal temper of heroic hearts,
Made weak by time and fate, but strong in will
To strive, to seek, to find, and not to yield.

I confided in Kevin, my assisting officer and dear friend who sat beside me at the funeral home. I always knew there was a chance Shawn may have been killed in the line of duty, but I never, ever imagined he would be taken down by illness. I asked Kevin if he thought the last three lines of this stanza would be fitting as the inscription on Shawn's headstone.

At first speechless and a little choked up, Kevin reflected, saying how well it encompassed Shawn's life and his work. He remarked how eloquently it described what they do in the military; the determination shared by soldiers and their comrades – blood pumping through their veins in symbiotic rhythm, forging ahead to achieve a common goal. If fate determined any of them should perish, their souls would live on… "and not to yield." Kevin then added, "If you don't use it, I will steal it for my own headstone."

I knew Shawn would embrace the lines I chose for his inscription, as we shared a love of Greek mythology. We both had a thirst to experience the history of Greece. In fact, the first night we met, we marveled how we had each booked trips to explore the Mediterranean after completing our degrees. Who knows? Maybe our paths had crossed before that day. Maybe we were destined to be together.

So on these days, when I wander around the graveyard, drawing in some peace and comfort, I feel that Shawn is sending me a message: "It is time to walk among the living."

Chapter Sixteen

The Thaw Begins

The days dragged on and my routines stayed the same, but I now found that I was recovering the ability to focus on other things that needed my attention.

I knew it was time to landscape my backyard, so I purchased the sod and the supplies I needed for building a deck.

Then, the military stepped in to help me. Thirty-two men and women arrived at my house one day in their physical training gear. They were happy to be away from work, out in the sunshine, and helping us build a new life. My heart swelled with pride, understanding that the military takes care of its own. Every man and woman exuded sheer concern for our situation and approached the day with a positive outlook.

Sometimes, I think Canadians lose sight of how lucky we are to live where we do, and to have the freedoms that come in a peaceful country. Military members have insight into the 'sheer luck' of where a person is born. To a military person, I think that cherishing days like this is a blessing. Shawn once explained to me why he had developed a positive outlook on life and why he looked at every beautiful, carefree day as a gift.

He talked about his tour in Bosnia in 1992. The tours were six months long, and each military member was entitled to a two-week leave midway through. They could choose to spend those two weeks traveling Europe or they could return home to their families. He decided to return home and told me how his choice played tricks with his mind, saying, "Imagine being in a war torn country for three months, being shot at by snipers while bombs are going off all around you. You have to constantly be alert and ready for danger. But, the next day you are back home in Canada, sitting in Don Cherry's, sipping a beer and eating wings. One loud noise in Don Cherry's could have you automatically jumping out of your seat, looking for cover, getting into fighting mode. Then two weeks later, you find yourself back in Bosnia at an outdoor restaurant with a C7 Assault Rifle strapped to your shoulder, hoping to get through your meal before insurgents terrorize the place. Relaxing could result in injury or death." He said, "It really screws with your head."

The military men and women lay the sod and worked hard. They joked and laughed with each other, and this made me feel alive for the first time in so long.

When the day was done, I didn't want them to leave and for the first time in over a year, I didn't feel sorry for myself; I felt *lucky*. They barely knew my husband. In fact, very few of them had actually worked with him, because he had gone immediately into the hospital after we were transferred to Edmonton. Yet they all wanted to help, and they did so with genuine joy.

I thought if each of us could take but *one* page from their book and gain enlightenment into our good fortune – *what a wonderful world it would be.*

Now that the sod was in and the deck was built, I started planning my garden. I went to a greenhouse and bought over thirty perennials, then spent most days digging in the dirt and planting. It was therapeutic to get into the earth and create something beautiful.

Neighbours finally moved in behind us and I was a bit leery about getting to know them, having heard rumours of the man being a bit of a hothead. But soon we were all the best of friends and he and his wife would often invite me and the kids over for drinks or a bonfire. I realized that I should never listen to rumours, because I may miss out on something truly wonderful.

Lexi also had a new friend, for the family had just purchased a male Staffordshire Terrier pup. They named him Lloyd, which suited him perfectly. He was a little ball of muscle with short stubby legs and a large triangular head. He was black and white and reminded me of a small cow. We would laugh at how cute he and Lexi were together. I think they thought they were mom and pup. They would chase each other around the yard, while pouncing and chewing on one another. Some days Lexi would come in the house resembling a pincushion for all of the puncture holes she had on her ears and head from Lloyd's razor sharp teeth, but she didn't seem to mind. Lloyd was the pup she never had, and if he got too carried away, she would quickly put him in his place.

The two of them got into the bad habit of chewing some of my new shrubs, and this was not cool! I had to replace a few of them and install wire fences. Not to mention the extra poop I had to pick up, because Lloyd preferred to do his business in our yard. I grumbled and cursed the two of them, but I wouldn't have traded a moment.

Many of my neighbours stepped in to help. I was overwhelmed with their kindness. In the beginning when we first moved in, Sandy from the street behind us, Kristi from two doors down, and Kim who lived only a few houses away, prepared a welcome basket filled with candles and linens. It seemed if ever I was feeling sad, all I had to do was step outside and one of my neighbours would provide what I needed.

I recalled when we first moved to the neighbourhood. Shawn was still in palliative care, but he was able to come home for brief visits by ambulance. These visits were difficult, especially for him. We had moved into our new house but he had never actually lived there, and we both realized he probably never would. I could see how this weighed on him. I walked with him around the house, showing him our progress, and I sensed he was filled with sadness and resentment. Who could blame him. All of the things he had worked for were being ripped away.

When our visit was over, I held his hand as he was hoisted into the ambulance, and stood there staring while the ambulance rounded the corner and disappeared out of sight. Filled with utter defeat, I sat down on the lawn and lowered my head in my hands, realizing this would most likely be the last time he came home. I rested there a moment consumed with grief… Soon Sandy and Kristi, who were on Kristi's front porch witnessing all of this, came over and sat beside me. They listened while I unloaded. I was able to freely share my fears, my anger, and my sadness. I still consider that day to be one of those unexpected miracles. I was feeling desperate and alone, and they were there to provide comfort.

From that day on, Sandy and I became very good friends. We both loved to exercise, so Sandy would take me on long bike rides in the river valley, and in return for kicking my butt, I took her to the pool and taught her how to swim effectively. I told her it was all about the breathing. We worked on her strokes and soon she was swimming thirty to forty minutes at a time. What I loved about Sandy was her ability to make light of situations. She was one of those rare people who are not afraid to say something off colour. Most people tip-toed around me, not wanting to add any stress, not daring to tell me about their problems – heaven forbid anyone have problems greater than mine! I often felt secluded, but not around Sandy and her husband Norbert. They faced tragedy head on, as they were able to find humour in almost any situation.

One time Sandy and I were swimming lengths. She was following behind me when I suddenly stopped at the wall and began to sob. Sandy took this in stride, also stopping at the wall.

She asked, "Are you all right?"

I explained, "The gentleman one lane over reminds me of how Shawn looked when he was very sick."

She looked over, no doubt noticing the frail man in his eighties, and without skipping a beat said, "Do you want me to ask him if he wants a date?"

Now we were both in tears, laughing hysterically! That is why I loved my friend Sandy.

Chapter Seventeen

When in Heaven...

Vivian said, "Shawn, we would love to show you around. That is, if you have the time?" She smiled, amused at her own wit.

Some things never change! he thought.

"Come! Climb in the canoe and follow us. You certainly don't need help paddling that boat, not with your physique. Ours is just over... Romeo," she bellowed, "where did you park that canoe?"

With an eye roll, he stepped aside to show her it was just behind him, pulled up on the shore.

She said, "Well, what are you two waiting for? Let's go then!"

Vivian rarely apologized. Rather, she would simply skip over her "brief" shortsightedness.

Shawn noticed Romeo's face and had to giggle. Romeo pursed his lips, scrunched his eyes, and threw his arms in the air, as if to say, "No sense starting something."

He wished Marie could be there to witness this. She would surely be in stitches. "Where are we going?" Shawn inquired.

"You ask a lot of questions, young man," was her reply.

"Yes, yes I do." he conceded. He shook his head, shut his mouth, and climbed in like he was told. He wondered where they could possibly be taking him. He hadn't felt this alive in so long. Then, realizing the irony in this, Shawn laughed to himself.

They pushed off, and he followed at a short distance. Shawn refused to miss any of the entertainment. Vivian and Romeo could break into another squabble at any moment. They paddled east around a mountain of such enormity, it overshadowed their presence at a magnitude that overwhelmed his senses. Shawn had been in the Rocky Mountains many times, and had experienced the grandeur of those magnificent rock structures, but this mountain was unique. He was certain that it continued below the water's surface with a mass equal to what was now visible above them. In fact, as he looked below the surface, it seemed to go on forever.

He thought, *when in heaven, I guess anything is possible.*

To have a mountain here was a gift in itself. The mountains in Canada were familiar territory for Shawn. He remembered how he would push his body to the point of exhaustion, just to reach the summit. He thought that nothing could equal the sensation of standing at the top of a mountain and viewing the expanse of the landscape below. The brisk air would cut through you, leaving you with the sensation of floating above the earth. It felt as though the wind, if strong enough, could carry you off the top. Mountains demand respect for all their beauty and magnitude. They allow you to trod upon them for pleasure, but they also make you realize how quickly one wrong move could leave you at their mercy.

He thought, if anything is Godlike, it is the mountains; they can provide such pleasure, but could also determine a person's ultimate demise.

Shawn thought back on how Marie almost determined his demise, the day he took her adventure training with the military.

*H*e was in Canmore, where one week of the year, the military would hold adventure training, including mountain climbing, canoeing, and kayaking. He had the bright idea that Marie might like to join him there, so he picked up the phone and called her.

"Marie, why don't you come to Canmore? You love the outdoors and we can do some hiking and canoeing together. It will be lots of fun!"

She was a trooper and it was her summer vacation, so she rushed out, bought some new hiking boots, and jumped in her Honda CRX. Six hours later, she arrived at the campsite in Canmore.

She was in decent shape, fairly athletic, and could swim a crazy number of lengths in the pool, so he thought that surely she would also be a great mountain climber.

It was the third day of adventure training and he had already climbed three mountains. His goal was to climb a mountain each day. Middle Sister Mountain was slated for the next day, and Rundle Mountain was to follow. He was pumped, especially because he would get to climb with his sweetie.

All evening, he built Marie up for the climb. He assured her it wouldn't be nearly as hard as Big Sister Mountain, and that she should have very little difficulty. Of course, she believed him. After all, he would never steer her wrong!

Goucher, their military guide, was a fanatic. He was a mountain climbing guru who had climbed all around the world, including a mountain called Jungfrau, which is one of the highest mountains in Switzerland. Marie knew this because she had also been to the top, but only by taking two trains! Goucher was like one of those energizer bunnies you see on television. Marie said this should have been her first clue that she was in over her head.

Everyone who knew Marie, knew that she was not a morning person. In fact, Shawn was certain Marie wanted to punch Goucher in the head for being so *perky* first thing in the morning.

They had their morning meal of military rations. Yummy! Marie really enjoyed that. Dehydrated cereal – just add water – and delicious. Her face was absolutely priceless. As she peered up over her bowl at Shawn, their eyes locked, and there was that silent understanding: he would pay for this later.

They stocked up on water and snacks, and were ready to tackle this mountain.

After the short drive to the base of Middle Sister, they pulled their gear out of the van, strapped on their backpacks, and set out. The mountain seemed relatively unthreatening at the start. In fact, the first stretch went very well. Marie was amazing and Shawn remembered thinking, "Was there anything this girl couldn't do?" She was out in front with the guide for the first two hours. He remembered how proud he was of her.

Then, she 'hit the wall.' She hadn't paced herself and he could see her frustration.

Shawn was starting to feel darts shooting from her eyes, and her words were becoming very short and to the point.

She began to get nasty, calling him names and cursing the very ground he walked on.

The transformation was frankly *quite frightening*. He had never seen this side of her.

She explained in no uncertain terms that she was a swimmer, and not a runner or a hiker, and how it was now clear to her that mountain climbing takes the development of certain muscle groups – which she did not possess.

Oh boy, he thought.

They started to take more breaks, and he was now carrying all the water.

When they got to the last stretch of the mountain they were faced with the hardest challenge yet – one hundred feet of shale. Marie was 'utterly impressed' now, because for every five steps they climbed, they would slide back three. This went on for about an hour.

He laughed now, thinking back on how she wanted to rip him a new one!

Then one of the military females decided to quit and he knew Marie would see this as her out. He knew she would have kept going out of sheer stubbornness, but since someone else had actually quit, this meant so could she.

He had to give her credit, because she had pushed herself to reach the top of the shale, thinking that was the summit, but when she got there she realized there was still about a hundred feet to go. That's when she threw her arms up in the air and told him where to go: "To the top without her!"

He considered trying to convince her to continue, but Goucher assured him that this would not be wise, or good for his health.

Needless to say, he and the group continued to the top and left Marie sitting there.

The top of the mountain was breathtaking and he wanted desperately to share it with her. He took out the camera and snapped some pictures at nine thousand and eighty-five feet in the air, while she sat on the ridge just one hundred feet below him. She told him later she had been quite content sitting there, watching the helicopters fly below her.

They laughed about it later – how she was *madder than a wet hen.*

It took them five hours to reach the top and four hours to descend the mountain.

Later that evening he and Marie were having dinner at a restaurant with the view of the Three Sister Mountains in the distance. He remembered asking if she was disappointed she had not reached the top.

She said she wasn't disappointed because she had reached the first peak and that was still a huge accomplishment. She never thought she would ever stand that high above the earth or push her body that hard.

As Shawn pensively gazed at the mountains, he smiled, thinking how that was definitely a 'glass half full' attitude. But, when he looked over at her, he saw that she had fallen asleep in her plate of spaghetti.

The next morning, for a fleeting moment, he thought about climbing Rundle Mountain. He even stupidly suggested she might like to join him. Daggers shot from her eyes. Wisely, he reconsidered, and suggested instead, "How about a nice, calm day of canoeing, a small hike up Sulphur Mountain, and then a gondola ride down, finishing with a hot tub?" Her eyes relaxed, and he smiled, realizing he would still be in this relationship when he returned home.

Chapter Eighteen

Coffee and a Lube

Have you ever had one of those mornings where you wonder how you got this far in life? You feel that someone should have thrown you off a cliff, thereby saving humanity from having to experience the most stupid person on the face of the earth? I've had one of those mornings. In fact, sometimes I think someone should have just put me to sleep, due to lack of brain activity.

I am referring to the day I made the nice young guy at the Jiffy Lube establishment shit his pants!

I was in the drive-thru getting my morning coffee. Remembering the Jiffy Lube place right next door, I decided I would pull around and get my oil changed as well.

I had rushed out of the house like most mornings, wearing white socks and these stupid black shoes that always slipped off the back of my heels, especially when I wore sport socks with them. The guy at the Jiffy Lube directed me into the garage bay and I was following his directions nicely, but when I tried to move my foot from the gas to the brake, the back of my shoe slipped off and got stuck between the mat and the gas pedal, pinning my foot down. At least, that is what I think happened. The truck engine roared and sped forwards towards this poor guy, and I envisioned myself hitting the young fellow square in the chest, killing him, and then continuing on to crash through the massive glass door behind him! Luckily, I was able to free my foot and slam on the brake, barely in time to stop the truck inches away from him.

Of course, everyone in the garage was staring at me, their mouths wide open in disbelief, including a young lady I had taught in Junior High. I wanted to shrink down into the seat and vanish from sight. I wanted to crawl into the hole I belonged in...but instead I began apologizing profusely, and the older gentleman actually said, "It happens!" Which was an outright lie, and I was certain he was planning on calling "Canada's Worst Drivers" as soon as I left, to sign up the next winner. The young man I had almost driven into, just smiled politely.

I humbly drank my coffee and got the hell out of there as quickly as possible, but before leaving, I apologized again to the young man for nearly taking his life.

He generously said, "No worries."

I told him I was *very worried*, and assured him that I was now only wearing my socks!

When I got home, I threw the damn shoes in the garbage and tried to settle my nerves.

I told myself that I would not speak of this to anyone. But, my defamatory personality almost always has me share these stories with people, so here I am sharing it with the world! This must be my way of punishing myself for my stupidity.

There were many days like this. I swear I was being tested.

Chapter Nineteen

More Surprises

Romeo and Vivian had become quite accomplished paddlers, and Shawn wondered how long they had been journeying around heaven together. He also wondered what was in store for him.

Where were they taking him?

As they reached the other side of the mountain, a new landscape unfolded. The gentle current carried them towards the shoreline, where he saw a beach filled with the finest white sand and a massive stairway made of uneven slabs of shale rising up to an open expanse of lush, velvet grass and trees of such grandeur. The sky above him was magically blue, and the pure, sweet air he breathed was intoxicating.

He searched his memory, but the landscape before him rivaled any storybook scene he could recall. Truly, he never thought he would experience anything so stunning.

They pulled the canoes on shore and he followed Romeo and Vivian up the shale stairs. There, in the distance under an enormous oak tree, he saw two women. They were lying flat on their backs, hands behind their heads, faces to the sky, and they were laughing and sharing stories.

Shawn thought one of them looked familiar, but had to move closer to recognize who she was. He felt warmth rise from his gut, then travel to his lips and spread across his face in a magnificent grin.

"JULIE!"

He recalled how devastated everyone had been. Initially, he had been driving home when he received the phone call. Vivian was calling him on his cell phone because she couldn't reach Marie. She wanted desperately to tell Marie before anyone else did.

He sped up quickly and rushed in the back door of the house, to find Marie doubled over with the phone still in her hand. One of her cousins had already told her. She just kept repeating, "NO... NOT JULIE! Not her!"

He remembered helping Marie to her feet and holding her tight in his arms while she wept.

Juliet was Marie's first cousin. She and Marie had been very close growing up; in fact, they were like sisters. They lived just one mile apart in the same small farming community along the North Saskatchewan River. Julie and her younger sister Lucille along with Marie and her older brother Mark were the youngest siblings of two large families. The four cousins were inseparable.

Shawn recalled Marie telling him how they would ride their bikes back and forth down that old country road and spend countless hours at each other's farms. They loved to explore the old outbuildings and barns, all the while inventing games to occupy their time. A few of their favourite activities included climbing into the rickety tree house at Julie and Lucille's farm, or rooting through the many rooms in the old pig barn at Mark and Marie's farm. She told him how they would be covered head to foot with hay from crawling in and out of the small spaces in the building, and how they loved playing in the hidden lofts.

Another of their favourite activities, were riding their bikes to the cemetery behind the old church and reading the headstones. He remembered the story she always told about the headstone of a gentleman named "Frank Sank". Suzanne would say, "Yes, Frank sank! He sank nine feet under." This never got old.

Marie always spoke of these memories with an endearing breathlessness. He almost felt envious of how magical her childhood sounded. It was simple and effortless, as a childhood should be.

As the cousins grew up, married, and had families of their own, they still remained close. They played co-ed volleyball and baseball together and socialized in the same circles.

The evening after Julie died, Shawn remembered how Marie ran a bath and lay there for hours, reminiscing and sobbing. He came in, only to offer her tea, sensing she needed to be alone in her thoughts. He remembered how helpless he felt, because there was nothing he could do to ease her pain.

Julie had two teenage girls and an adoring husband. Julie and Larry had the kind of marriage many people wish for. They were best friends. Even when they were apart, they were conversing throughout the day by phone.

It happened one week before Julie's forty-first birthday. Initially, Marie thought it must have been a car accident that took her since her death was so sudden, but then she learned that Larry had rushed Julie to the hospital because she had serious flu-like symptoms, including an elevated fever and vomiting. Within twenty-four hours she was gone. Later, they discovered she had contracted meningitis, and still to this day, no one is certain where she came in contact with the disease.

And here she was – beneath that giant oak tree.

Shawn practically yelled her name, no longer able to contain his joy, and he threw himself down on his knees before her, just as she sat up, and they hugged tightly.

"Shawn, my God, it's so good to see you," she said, finally letting go. "I have so many questions. I don't even know where to begin!"

"Shawn, you remember Jocelyn… Oh, I'm sorry. That's right. Jocelyn was already gone when you met Marie."

Half out of breath, he held out his hand, "Hello Jocelyn. It's fantastic to finally meet you. This whole day has been simply amazing! I'm completely overwhelmed! In my wildest dreams, I never, ever thought I would meet the rest of Marie's family."

Then Jocelyn joked, "Believe me, I understand your bewilderment. It is a lot to take in. I'm still trying to figure out how I made it to this place!" and she laughed.

He giggled. "Marie told me about your sense of humour. Wow! This is amazing. Just bloody amazing," and he hugged her. Then he poured on the charm, "Jocelyn, I knew you were a looker, but no one warned me that you would take my breath away!"

"Marie certainly picked right this time," she said. "They told me you were smart, but I had no idea you were brilliant!" Then turning to Romeo and Vivian, she said, "I like this guy."

Vivian rolled her eyes, "Oh brother!"

Shawn was still in awe. As a man of many words, he added, "I just can't believe I'm here talking to all of you. First Marie's dad, then her cousin, and now her sister!"

"Best for last," Jocelyn joked.

Chapter Twenty

Sharing Stories

Shawn sat sharing stories with Julie and Jocelyn for most of the day. He described Jarryd and Cole first by saying, "They are the spitting image of me." Then he told them how each of the boys shared some of his interests; for example, Jarryd loved to play soccer. "He is a goalkeeper, just like I was. He also loves to build things and take them apart piece by piece. He is mathematical and absorbs factual information like a sponge. I'm sure he is going to be an engineer."

Shawn continued, "Cole is an artist. He loves to draw just like me. He is also very musical. He plays piano by ear. Marie always laughs, saying how he must have inherited that talent from Uncle Norman, because she didn't have a musical bone in her body, but I would disagree with her, saying she could sing like an angel."

"Sing?" both Julie and Jocelyn chimed in.

"Yes, she would often sing to me in the car. I'm glad she felt comfortable enough to sing in front of me. She was really very shy about it."

Julie and Jocelyn gave each other a sideways glace, as though they shared an inside joke. But Jocelyn just couldn't let this one go. "You really were mesmerized, my dear. As far as I remember, there were very few members of our family who could sing. Mind you, Dad could always sing and so could Norman, but…Marie? That is interesting, to say the least." Then she shook her head and said, "I think *you*, my dear, were deafened by love!"

Shawn giggled. "Maybe," he said, "but when I was away, I couldn't wait to call and hear her voice. I called every chance I got. It tore me apart when I had to leave her. Part of me was always there. I couldn't wait for the day I would retire from the military and spend the rest of my life making it up to her. I only had five years left, you know. I went back to college through the military to obtain a career in Biomedical Engineering, and once I was finished my service it was my intent to work in a hospital close to home fixing medical equipment. But life doesn't always work out the way you have planned."

Jocelyn said, "Tell me how you two met."

"We met at a military party when I first transferred to the base in Edmonton. My wife and I had split about six months earlier and I was trying to get back on my feet again. I was busy taking medical courses and I knew very few people in Edmonton – only the ones I had done training or tours with."

Marie and her friends had planned a girls' night. They intended to visit the various pubs in the University area and get very drunk. They started at a little English pub, sharing stories and having a few drinks…when Stacey entered.

Stacey was a delightful pretty little blonde with big green eyes that sparkled. She also had this infectious laugh, and she had most certainly started on the drinks early! Marie had never met her before, but she liked her instantly. Stacey told her friend Sandra how she had just come from a friend's house where she had met some military guy and now she really, really wanted to go party with him.

In fact, she said he had invited all of them to the party. They blew her off for a while, but she would not take "no" for an answer.

Next thing they knew, they were going to a party at the military base. Marie said she was a little nervous, because it was late in the evening, and they had all heard stories about those military types: testosterone bearing, twelve sandwich eating, gun toting, hormone raging, alcohol driven, party animals!

They finally gave in by responding, "Well okay, but we will keep the cab running."

As they entered the barracks and climbed the stairs to the second floor, Marie was thinking, "Four girls showing up at a party at ten-thirty in the evening with a bunch of drunken military men – this is a really bad idea." But they were already there, so she decided they might as well check it out.

She told Shawn later, "The things you do for your friends!"

It wasn't so bad. The barracks were laid out like an apartment complex with four floors. The party was on the second floor, and everyone was in the hallway. There were couches and chairs lining both sides of the hallway and a stereo had been set up at the back wall.

Walking in was a bit unnerving, because a bunch of heads turned, and she said she could literally see the hazy, alcohol-induced thought patterns register across most of their foreheads… "Four desperate females that want to get laid." They couldn't have been farther from the truth, at least as far as Marie was concerned, but who could blame them for thinking that. It really did look bad!

As she sat down, her attention was instantly drawn to the Newfoundlander, surrounded by a group of inebriated men. They were singing along to obscene songs, while he played the guitar. They were actually quite comical and Shawn remembered how a crowd had gathered around, egging them on.

Stacey was quick in pursuit of her love interest, so Marie and Sandra quietly opened their beers across from a bunch of people they didn't know.

Low and behold, some really drunk guy came over and said to Marie: "Hey, you're cute; I bet you girls are here to get lucky. Well, it's your lucky day because I am willing and able!"

Marie laughed out loud, promptly finishing his statement, "and drunk," then proceeded to tell him about that frosty day in hell we have all been waiting for! This didn't seem to register so she lashed out again with a few more nasty retorts. And with a glazed, rather vacant look he stumbled away to the next unsuspecting victim. He was a good looking guy, but that quickly diminished with the first words out of his mouth.

At that moment, Marie was thinking how many ways she would make Stacey pay for this.

Shawn continued, "I noticed her right away. She was attractive and could handle herself. It took some courage, especially after I saw her shoot the last guy down in flames, but I took the seat beside her. We engaged in conversation and talked most of the evening. I gave her my phone number and asked her to call me for coffee sometime. She did! The rest is history..."

Jocelyn's eyes filled with tears. As she stood up, she took Shawn by the hand and led him to a serene little section of paradise tucked away in the trees. It was a small pond you might see in the movies, where one could spend an entire day fishing or swimming with friends. Jocelyn explained how she had named it 'Mystery Pond' after the pond down by the river on the farm, as the similarities between the two were eerily familiar.

Shawn, somewhat bewildered by Jocelyn's tears, sat down and quietly listened as she reminisced about her life.

"All five of us kids loved to go down to the pond. Life was so simple then. Mark and Norman would clear the snow to make a skating rink; Marie would help them flood the ice, hauling buckets of water from the house. When the ice was ready, they would strap on their skates and spend hours horsing around. Marie would try to dazzle them with her fancy pirouettes, urging them to try. Meanwhile, Mark and Norman would be shooting a ball around with hockey sticks."

Jocelyn explained, "Suzanne, Norman, and I were much older than the younger two. In fact, Suz and I had moved out by then and Norman left not long after. We were actually more like two separate families growing up, for the large seven-year age difference that separated us older three from Mark and Marie. As I think back, this place was meaningful to all of us. I remember it was Suzanne and I who named the pond, for it had appeared mysteriously one summer when I was eleven years old. I remember the county had begun to excavate the river valley that summer for a pipeline that was to run under the river. As the gravel was cleared and pulled back in huge mounds, the river water filtered through the gravel bed along the shore, and the water that came through was crystal clear. Once the big machines were finished at the end of the summer, Suzanne and I decided to go exploring. Because the riverbank was so densely treed, we couldn't see anything from the road. and we actually had to climb over the enormous gravel mounds to see what they had done. We were astonished to discover that the river bank had been transformed into a quaint little pond and it seemed to have appeared out of nowhere. That's why we called it Mystery Pond. The water was clear and the digging of gravel had created a long narrow peninsula with all of the driftwood piled up. It was stunning!"

Then Jocelyn explained the reason for her tears: "If only things could have been different once I grew up. More importantly, I wish I could take back the mistakes I've made in my life and start over from when we were innocent kids. I certainly would have made better choices. Marie probably told you about my addiction? I let alcohol consume my life. I rarely saw what was right in front of me and I hurt the people that I love. I have many regrets."

Shawn consoled her, "It sounds like you were in pain. I hope you don't mind, but Marie shared a little about your illness. She said you had everything going for you. You were funny, smart, beautiful…but rarely happy. She said alcohol played a large part in your life spinning out of control, but she never believed that was the source of your illness."

Jocelyn smiled slightly, "My sister is a smart girl. I agree with her. I believe that alcohol was only the crutch I used. I often fell into dark, debilitating depressions and sometimes they went on for days. It seemed I was never truly happy."

Shawn continued, "Marie told me she wanted to help, but didn't know how. She believes you are now at peace and this makes her truly happy. Jocelyn, you can't change what happened in your life, but you have to forgive yourself. It sounds like you suffered from extreme depression." Then he asked, "Did you have a support system? Someone you could talk to?"

Jocelyn was silent for a moment, and then replied, "The family tried to help. Mom and Dad, who often spent their winters in Arizona, eventually checked me into a highly-respected treatment facility. I went through the program and I was clean for several months. Once I recognized my problem, I attended Alcoholics Anonymous almost daily. My intentions were always the best: I would be sober for months, but I always surrendered to the bottle. It was as though I thought the bottle could erase my pain. I was a tortured soul. I always had a strained relationship with my mother. We just never saw eye to eye. I realize now that she was also suffering from issues of abandonment. We have shared many conversations here, and made up for lost time. I always believed she was against me, but the truth was she didn't know how to reach me. Instead of being sympathetic, she became frustrated. We butted heads something fierce."

Jocelyn continued, "Now that I think back, I was always a lot of trouble – even when I died. My request was not simple, based on deep seeded fears. I didn't want to be put in the ground because of my claustrophobia and my fear of spiders. I also made Larry and the girls promise not to cremate my remains, because I had been burned so badly. Even in death, I was a royal pain in the butt!" She giggled. "Even so, they respected my wishes and found a cemetery in Arizona that would encrypt my remains in an airtight wall casket."

Shawn couldn't help but laugh and appreciate her sense of humour.

"Did Marie tell you the story of how I was burned?" Jocelyn asked.

"Sort of, but I'd like to hear your version," he replied.

Jocelyn began, "Larry and I had been married only a few months. We packed up the truck and camper and drove out to our favourite lake. One of Larry's friends had come with us. On our first night, we must have left the propane open on the stove; I think it had been on all night. The next morning, our friend left to use the outhouse and I was still in my bunk. Larry had just gotten up. He removed a cigarette from the pack, flicked the wheel on the lighter, and that is when the propane ignited! Our only saving grace was that our friend had left the door on the camper slightly ajar. The force of the explosion kicked the door open, releasing the gas and flames, and then slammed the door shut with a tremendous bang. My worst burns were the ones on my hands, because that doorknob was surely the temperature of the sun, but still I pulled, turned, and kicked, fighting to get out.

"Believe me when I say I wished I had died that day, to escape the pain that followed. I was burned on seventy-five percent of my body – all second and third degree burns. I had been wearing flimsy baby doll pajamas and the fabric melted to my skin. Larry was wearing jeans and a cotton shirt, which provided some protection; therefore he was not as badly burned. He spent one month in hospital while I spent three. You wouldn't wish this kind of pain on your worst enemy. Every day I begged my family to let me die. I remember telling my daughters how hard it was to recover from those burns. And although the physical recovery was terrible, the mental recovery was much worse.

"My self-esteem had been low before, but now it seemed nothing could save me. At least my face wasn't badly burned; however, the scars on my body were hideous! I was able to cover most of my skin with clothing, but any time my scars were visible, adults and children would stare. I felt like 'that car wreck you come across and just can't turn away from.' To me, my body was a smoldering mess. Maybe you can understand how that feels?"

"Oh Jocelyn, I am so sorry you had to go through that," Shawn sympathized.

"A few years later," Jocelyn reflected, "Larry and I were blessed with an adorable baby girl. We named her Trinity. She was the most beautiful thing I had ever seen. Her tiny fingers and toes were splendidly perfect in every way. I marveled that we had created this tiny angel, and I watched her grow. Two years later we were blessed with another baby girl, and we named her Jessica. If there is one thing I will never regret, it is having those two girls. They brought incredible joy to my life and I loved them with all my heart. Now they have gone on to have their own families. Jessica named her second child 'Jocelyn'. She chose Lailani for her middle name, which means 'heavenly flower'. Isn't that marvelous? My heart swells with pride when I think of the women my daughters have become."

Jocelyn continued, "When the girls were five and seven years old, Larry and I separated. It was more than I could bear. I tried to run away from my problems, and the girls and I relocated in Arizona permanently. I thought I could hide and drown my sorrows, but moving there was a terrible mistake, for I was more isolated than ever before. Worse, I felt that my family gave up on me. I guess they thought 'tough love' would be best. They hoped that if I hit rock bottom, I would pick myself up and want to stay sober. Although their intentions were good, this was the worst thing they could have done. I had felt abandoned by loved ones my whole life, so in my mind this confirmed all that I ever believed. Now I was really alone, and my best friend became the bottle."

"Oh Jocelyn, I am so sorry," Shawn said, consoling her.

"The worst part was," Jocelyn added, "I felt I was always judged for my choices, but alcohol had been the catalyst for so much pain in my family's history, leaving a path of destruction throughout several generations. At least my girls saw clearly what it did to our family, and consequently have never touched a drop. They watched how I was tortured by it, and how it robbed them of their childhood. They learned from our mistakes and that makes me very proud."

Chapter Twenty-One

Vivian

Shawn saw Vivian walking towards him. She complained that everyone was stealing his attention, and asked if they could walk awhile. Now it was her turn. A smile spread across Shawn's face, knowing that this was Vivian's way of saying how happy she was to see him again.

She appeared a bit uncomfortable, and began unloading the thing that weighed heavily on her heart. "I have such regret that I left Marie and the boys at this time in their lives. I was thinking only of myself, and it was selfish not to treat my breast cancer."

Shaking his head, Shawn replied, "Marie only wanted what you wanted. She knew you needed to be with Romeo and she would never have asked you to stay for her. She's a big girl. Her only regret is that she wasn't there to hold your hand through it all. She never wanted you to experience cancer treatments. She understood your fears. Quality of life is so much more important than quantity. Although she misses you every day, she knows you are at peace. She had you with her for forty-two years. You two had a connection with each other that many people would kill for. She told me that you were the 'voice of reason.' Funny, but the priest at your funeral mocked Marie when she called you that in her eulogy, and Marie was angry, saying that you deserved that title as much as any deity."

Vivian laughed, drawing comfort from Shawn's words.

He continued to set her heart at ease. "That's how much she admired you. She loved you for your curt sarcasm and unique sense of humour, for your ageless wisdom, and for your unshakable strength. Her deepest wish was for those qualities to rub off on her. Every day she becomes stronger, it is because of you. Your words ring true in how she lives her life, and your love is still with her. Don't spend another moment in regret, Vivian, for your daughter only wishes you peace and love."

As Shawn looked at Vivian, he could feel the weight lifting from her. The deep creases around her eyes relaxed, and her shoulders fell. Tears of joy streaked her face and she said, "Thank you Shawn!"

"My pleasure; now let's enjoy our day." They sat together, looking towards the earth, watching…

Chapter Twenty-Two

Jarryd

Jarryd tried not to think of his dad, but nearly everything in his room was a reminder. There was the dragon perched atop his dresser that his dad had bought for him while on tour in Croatia. It had been intricately painted with bold detail and mounted on a wooden platform.

Jarryd remembered how his dad had grinned proudly, pulling the dragon out of his bag and handing it to him. Shawn knew Jarryd would love the gift and could barely contain his excitement.

Jarryd's eyes had grown wide with wonder and he couldn't wait to hold it. It was the coolest gift he had ever seen! Dragons were his favourite thing in the whole world. Though he had been only four years old at the time, his dad had trusted him with this delicate ceramic statue that could so easily have been dropped and broken. His dad explained how it was not a toy, but a keepsake to be kept on a shelf, only taken down occasionally to admire.

His dad's smile was as clear as yesterday. Jarryd loved the dragon, but it was his dad's smile that had been the best part of the gift.

Jarryd continued to scan his room. He stopped to focus on the top shelf in his closet. There sat the tool shed he and his dad had built for a grade three Science Fair project. He remembered Mom being rather pushy about them doing the project together. But thinking back, he was sure glad she was.

He and his dad had spent hours in the garage cutting, nailing, and gluing the pieces in place. They spray painted the walls and roof grey, and later added shingles and finer details with a small paint bush and black marker. Jarryd remembered how they had made small replicas of simple and compound machines to put inside the shed. He thought about the Science Fair morning when he and his dad had walked into the school and how so many kids had come to admire their work. Jarryd felt enormous pride and a huge sense of accomplishment. Most importantly, they had done it together!

Later that year, he and his dad had also taken on a much larger project. Jarryd smiled, thinking about how his dad got a bit carried away while building the tree house. Jarryd thought about how his dad never went into anything halfway. One of his favourite sayings was: "If you're going to do a job, do it right!"

Their property in Ontario included a half-acre of forested land at the back of the house. Together they chose three rather large, widely-spread trees in which to perch the tree house. Needless to say, by the time it was finished, it was more like a small house. His dad installed windows and even built a fancy ramp with a rope attached so that they could climb up. He made a trap door and hung a swing underneath. It was quite extravagant! His mom had laughed and said that they might need to check into getting a permit, it was so big.

Although he was only six years old, his dad still had him out there helping. He remembered being more of a hindrance than a help. His dad would give him directions, and Jarryd would do the exact opposite. For example, his dad told him to stay on the side of the tree house where the boards were already securely nailed down. But because he didn't listen, Jarryd slid on one of the loose boards and fell off the platform. He landed on his butt, his leg pinned by the board, but luckily nothing was broken.

His dad frantically scooped Jarryd up in his arms and hurried towards the house to check out any injuries. His mom saw them coming from the kitchen window and ran outside, yelling, "What happened?" When she heard that he fell, she shouted, "Oh, my God! I knew this would happen. Why weren't you watching him?"

His dad replied, "I told him not to stand on the loose boards..." but stopped mid-sentence. There was no point in trying to explain. Jarryd knew his mom was not impressed, and he remembered feeling worse about his dad getting in trouble than about hurting himself.

Jarryd was thinking how insignificant that pain was, compared to the pain he felt now. God, how he missed his dad!

Curling his fists until his knuckles turned white, Jarryd punched his pillow repeatedly. All of the pent up anger came out of him in hot tears. Why him? Why did everyone have a dad, but him? How could he possibly go his entire life without seeing his dad's smile or hearing his kind voice? Who would help him through difficult times? Who would understand him?

He could barely catch his breath as each sob assaulted his body with more force. Pain ripped through his core with such intensity he thought he would surely split in half.

Then he remembered the long talks he and his dad would have during time-outs. His dad would go on and on, and Jarryd would eventually tune him out. He laughed out loud remembering this. During those talks he dreaded being held captive, and would start squirming while his mind wandered off somewhere else. He wondered if his dad had known he was being tuned out?

What he wouldn't give for one of his dad's long-winded talks right now.

His dad always took the time to console him. He could relate, telling stories of when he was a boy, how he had experienced the same feelings of frustration, and how he got into the same sorts of trouble. He seemed to understand exactly how Jarryd's mind worked. His mom never seemed to 'get' the ways boys think. "Dumb girls," Jarryd thought, and giggled to himself, because he knew his dad would find this funny.

Just then, Lexi walked into the room and jumped on the bed. Her warm, sloppy tongue licked Jarryd's face repeatedly, lapping away the salty tears. Jarryd felt better, connected somehow. He put his arms around her big head and just knew that everything would be all right. He put his hand on Lexi's enormous chest and rubbed the white patch of hair.

His mom walked in the bedroom. She could see he had been crying. "Sweetheart, what's wrong?" she asked.

"I miss him so much," Jarryd blubbered through his tears.

"Me too," she said tenderly.

"Lexi is such a sweetie. She came to me and made me feel better."

"You know your dad wanted us to have her. I'm glad he talked me into getting her. I think he knew we would always feel protected with Lexi. Animals seem to know when you're hurting, and they bring such comfort. I don't know what we would have done without her."

"Mom, maybe Dad's spirit went into her."

"Maybe. That is such a comforting thought. Jarryd, your dad's spirit is always with us."

"It's just so unfair."

"I know, sweetheart, but your dad would want you to be happy. Whenever you feel sad, just hug Lexi; she'll make you feel better. I'm always here for you too. You know that, right?"

Chapter Twenty-Three

Cole

Raya guided Shawn to a bench in the garden, where they could watch Marie interact with Cole. Raya knew this was something he needed to see.

Cole was in the bathtub, and Marie sat on the floor next to him. He was telling her how he felt responsible for Shawn's death.

Marie gasped, "How could you say that, Cole? You could never be responsible!"

"I caused him to have stress, and that is why he died of stomach cancer."

"No sweetie, this was hereditary. That means this disease was passed down through the family. You had nothing to do with the cancer."

Cole continued, "And I told him I hated him one time when we were fighting. I never got to take that back!"

"Oh honey," she said. "I remember saying that to my parents when I was young. We say things sometimes when we are angry, but trust me; he knew you didn't mean it. He always knew how much you loved him."

Through sobs, Cole asked, "How do you know?"

"Because he left you a letter."

"He did?"

"Yes, he did. I was going to save it for when you are older, but if you want to hear it now, I can read it to you."

"Yes Mom, please let me hear it."

Marie went into the bedroom and came back a few minutes later with the letter.

She told him, "Your dad was too weak to write it himself, so I wrote his words while he spoke. We had to write it in two parts, because he was very sick and needed to rest, but these were his words."

August 8, 2008

The Letter-Part 1

Dear Cole,

Reading this now, you're much older. Through no choice of my own, I missed years of your life. I know deep inside of me that you will become a great man. There is no doubt in my mind. I hope you don't smoke. All I can do is hope! I hope you are good to people and they will be good to you. Trust me!

Always keep smiling and keep your attitude of travel and laughing.

You were always smart in school. I don't know if you get it from your mother or me, or maybe Jarryd. Who knows? You can be anything you want to be; just believe in yourself like I believe in you. I always told your mom you'd be okay.

August 9, 2008

Part 2

The love that you express to other people is very positive, and every day people like to be with you. Keep your love strong and show them you can be strong.

I love you always,

Dad

Shawn turned to Raya, his face soaked in tears. "I died three days later. Cole was seven years old. I had so much more to say to him…"

Marie barely made it through the letter. Cole's body slumped in defeat and he drew his knees in tight to his chest, longing for comfort, while huge tears rolled down his cheeks. His sobs came from deep in his chest. Shawn wanted desperately to pick him up and hold him in his arms, for he felt his son's pain with every gut wrenching sob.

Shawn could see Marie desperately searching in her mind for a way to lift the weight of the world from Cole's little shoulders.

If only she could make him laugh, it might take away some of his sadness.

Then Marie started to work her magic. "Cole, do you remember how Daddy loved his cars? Do you realize he bought eleven cars in the eleven years we were married? Isn't that ridiculous? He used to trade them like underwear!"

Cole giggled and his face brightened. "That's funny Mommy!"

"Yep, he would frustrate me to no end with those cars. I would think he had finally found the car of his dreams, and the next thing I knew he would be on the internet researching for a new one. Remember the last one, the Subaru WRX sports car? I still have the little toy replica in my room. Your dad bought it because it was an exact copy of his WRX. Cole, I know he would love for you to have it."

Cole's eyes widened. "Really?" he said, squealing with delight.

"Remember how you, Daddy, and Jarryd would cruise around town with the sunroof open and that darn stereo blasting? It's no wonder any of you have any hearing left at all! In fact, that little model car has a stereo exactly like the one in the WRX. Let me show you."

She left the room and returned with the model car in her hands. Then she showed him how to open the small doors. The lights flashed and the stereo thumped, playing the loud upbeat music.

Cole laughed. "Mommy, wasn't that the car you backed into?"

Shawn thought, *that little devil, Marie had known that Cole would take the bait.*

Playing along, Marie sheepishly lowered her head in shame. "Sure was." But then, she couldn't contain her laughter, and encouraged Cole to tease her like always.

"Mom, weren't we late for the Santa Claus parade? You were really mad at Jarryd and me for fighting," he reminisced quite proudly.

"I sure was, and I didn't even look behind me. Remember how I hastily threw the truck in reverse and backed out of the garage? It wasn't until I heard the sound of crushing metal that it dawned on me... Your dad had left his car outside! The truck bumper made contact, actually raising the car clear off the ground. I was mortified!" She twisted and contorted her face to show Cole how she must have looked. "Remember how I went running into the house sobbing, and I told your dad, 'I wrrrrecked your carrrrr!' BAAAAAH! WAAAAAA!"

Cole was really howling now.

Then, she demonstrated his dad's look of horror, and how his body had stiffened, fear flashing across his face at first in disbelief, but as her sobbing got louder, he pictured his 'pride and joy' crushed beyond all recognition.

She told Cole, "I knew your dad was furious, but he held it all inside, and he didn't yell at me. It took everything he had, but your dad in a very quiet voice simply stated through his trembling lips, "It's only a car. It's only a car..." as if trying to convince himself.

Cole asked, "Mommy, remember how he grabbed his cigars and stomped outside?"

"Yes," she answered, "and I ran into the bedroom, threw myself down on the bed, and bawled my eyes out! BAAAAA! WAAAAAA!"

Cole was laughing so hard now that tears were running down his cheeks. Still choking in laughter, he said, "I remember how Daddy said he needed his cigars!"

Meanwhile, up in heaven, Raya and Shawn were laughing so hard they almost fell off the bench.

Marie continued, "Yes, he was pacing around the outside of the house, intensely puffing on his cigar. I am sure every time he walked by the twisted remains of what used to be his baby, there were a few choice words directed at me. Did you know that later, your dad took both vehicles to the body shop to have them fixed? The guy at the auto body shop took one look at the car and gasped, 'What happened?'

"Your dad replied, 'My wife!'"

"The guy just shook his head, no doubt feeling every bit of your dad's pain." Marie continued, "Your dad and that guy must have had a good old vent about 'women drivers.' But I think your dad forgave me, because he asked the guy to fix my truck bumper once he was finished fixing the 'entire side panel' of his precious car. Your dad was a great guy! He told me he didn't want the bumper to be a constant reminder of what I had done to his car. Anyway Cole, this little model car is yours if you want it."

Marie could tell he was feeling much better now. She helped him out of the tub, wrapped him in a big, fluffy towel, and gave him a huge bear hug. "This one is from me and your dad," she said.

Chapter Twenty-Four

Making Connections

"Julie," Shawn asked, "do you ever watch what is going on with Larry and the girls? Have you ever let them know that you are present?"

"Yes, Shawn. I have made myself known a few times," she replied. "For example, I like to play with the garage door at the house, and I like to appear in photographs of the girls. I am very fortunate because my girls and Larry are spiritually aware. They are open to my presence... I often appear as orbs of light, in their pictures. In fact, Larry shared some of these photographs with Marie, and at first she tried to explain the bizarre circles of light and blurred segments of colour as something that happened in the developing process. But then, she noticed all of the photographs had these orbs of light. They were around the girls in every photograph, and they were abundant."

Then, Julie inquired, "Shawn, have you ever watched or made yourself known to Marie or the boys?"

"Yes, I have. In fact, I watched Jarryd catch a huge spring salmon just off the shore of Vancouver Island. He saw me, but no one else did."

"Ten months after I had passed, Marie opened her email to find a message. It was a special offer sponsored by the military to travel by train anywhere in Canada. Marie and I had spoken about travelling by train through the Rockies, but we never had the opportunity… If Marie had learned nothing else during the past two years, she learned that 'life is too short' and you have to take advantage of opportunities when they are given. This was the opportunity of a lifetime and the boys would love it! Without giving it a second thought, she checked into the details and booked three seats for the middle of July."

"My good friend Victor was living on Vancouver Island with his family. He had begun his career as a doctor in the military, but he was now an ER doctor at one of the hospitals on the island. We were very close friends; in fact, I had asked him and his wife to be Cole's Godparents. Marie thought this trip would be the perfect chance for Cole to get to know them better as they had moved to the Island when our boys were very young."

"When Marie called Vic to tell him the news, he immediately insisted that Marie and the boys stay with them. Because the trip would only be four days including travel, she accepted. Vivian had this saying: '*Company are like fish. They start to smell after three days.*' Marie always remembered that."

"They spent twenty-four hours on the train, only stopping once in Jasper. Since they were travelling economy class, they had to sleep in their seats, which was very uncomfortable, but no one complained. There were plenty of other children on the train and the boys kept busy playing cards and electronic games, visiting the viewing cars, and watching movies."

"The scenery was as breathtaking as Marie had imagined. In fact, while she sat in the dining car, the conductor announced that they should watch for some world famous waterfalls. She just happened to have her camera and was able to snap the most amazing photo of the Cascade Waterfalls. Marie no longer took these rare moments for granted, something as simple as being at the right place at the right time."

"They arrived early the next morning and were greeted at the Vancouver Ferry by Victor's wife Kirsten and their three girls. Cole was excited about having so many 'sisters'. He counted them saying, 'Including Amber, Jasmine, and Lexi, I have six sisters.' He was very proud of this fact."

"The trip was amazing. They toured the entire island, stopping at several beaches where the kids buried each other in the sand and collected various sea creatures. Of course, they had to release the sea life in their buckets before they left. Cole was not happy about this. He wanted to keep them to bring home, but eventually was convinced that sea creatures could not possibly survive away from their environment."

"Jarryd, like me, loves to fish. He could fish from sun-up to sun-down, every day of the year – must be something in the blood. He is passionate about fishing, and when Victor learned this, he booked a fishing charter on the ocean. The boat could only accommodate four passengers, so Vic decided to go with Marie and our boys."

"Jarryd was captivated by the fishing boat captain and asked him every question he could think of. He was especially impressed with all of the gear and helped the captain set up the rods and secure them to the boat. The captain taught Jarryd how to watch carefully for any signs of a nibble on the lines."

"Marie seemed to be getting more action on her side, so she asked Jarryd to switch with her. She said having him there would surely bring them all luck. However, the day started dragging as no one was getting a single bite. The boys' excitement began fading. Jarryd was now slouching in his seat and getting very impatient."

"Marie reminded him they could be at home instead of out here on the ocean, and tried to cheer Jarryd up by pointing out the beautiful scenery. About this time, they saw a bald eagle flying overhead and Vic was able to snap an amazing photo of this magnificent creature. This interested Jarryd, so he started paying more attention to his surroundings. He began scanning the rocks and looking out across the crystal water…"

"When he saw me, his eyes filled with tears. He waved and I waved back, smiling at him with pride. Marie said, 'What it is sweetie?"

"Jarryd said, 'You won't believe me, Mom, but I just saw Dad over there,' pointing to the shore. She didn't know what to say…she sat frozen, scanning the shoreline, searching…longing to see me for herself."

"Victor broke the silence by saying, 'Your dad is here, Jarryd. He is always with you. I know it in my heart.'"

"Marie's eyes filled with tears and the fishing boat captain joined their conversation, sharing a story about his mother. He told them that when his aunt died, his mother had known even before receiving the call because his aunt came to his mother the night before in a dream, telling her she loved her."

"The captain assured Jarryd, 'You're not crazy. Your dad is watching. Our loved ones come to us when we need them. He wouldn't want to miss this moment for the world. It is something special you and he shared, and something that will always connect you.' Marie was baffled! She hadn't expected this man, a stranger, to shed light on the situation."

Shawn told Julie, "My dear friend Victor, my wife, my sons, and this total stranger were brought together to share stories about faith and love. How wonderful!" Then he asked, "Julie, this man was a messenger from God, wasn't he?"

"Yes," she nodded. "There are more messengers of God than we could ever imagine."

The conversation on the boat was interrupted when Jarryd's line jerked. The captain was up on his feet and Jarryd snapped into reality. Adrenaline raced through his veins and he was ready to pull in his fish. Sure enough, he caught a twenty-one pound Spring Salmon. This monster wore him out! It fought and pulled at his line, and the captain instructed him when to let him run and when to reel with all his might.

"Keep the line tight," he advised, "but you also have to let him run, to tire him out."

Jarryd's smile stretched from ear to ear. He was in his element. He was a true fisherman and Shawn beamed along with him. Shawn smiled in heaven, bathing in Jarryd's glory. At the same time, regret bit at the back of his throat. Why? Why was he here and not there, sharing in his family's joy? He so wanted to be with them.

When they finally brought the enormous fish aboard and netted him, he flopped furiously around the deck. Jarryd had to whack him on the head with the hammer. He hit him cautiously the first time, and the fish went crazy and thrashed even more. Out of the net now, the salmon flopped under the seat where they were sitting.

Marie laughed at how ridiculous they looked as they lifted their feet, allowing the fish to burrow itself in the space beneath the bench.

The captain told Jarryd, "You have to hit him hard enough to knock him unconscious." He grabbed the fish, hooking his fingers in its gills, while Jarryd smacked the fish harder. Marie knew this took a lot of courage and she held her breath, grimacing as she watched him bat the fish on its head. But finally, the fish stopped moving, and she let the air escape from her mouth.

You couldn't wipe the smile off Jarryd's face all day. He had reeled in the big one, and he had done it with his dad there as his witness.

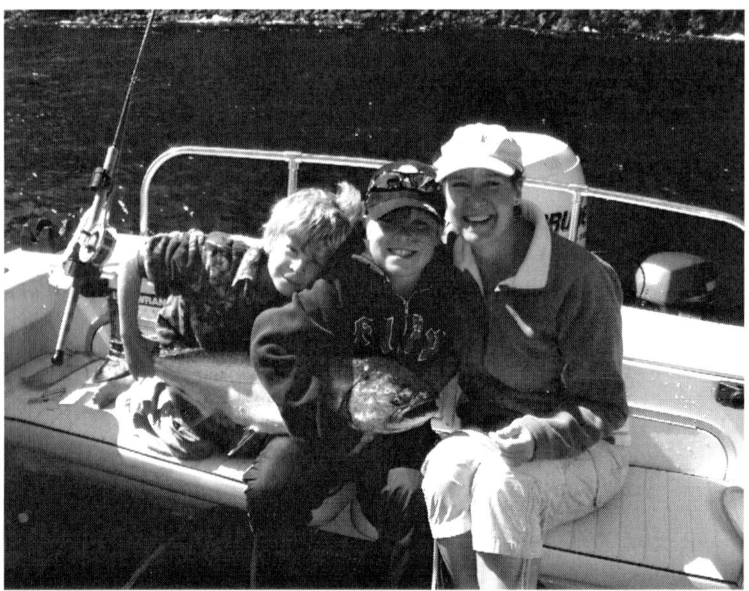

"I am so proud of you son!" As Shawn spoke these words aloud, he realized Julie was staring at him while he was off in another world.

Shawn told Julie how Cole and Jarryd talked to his picture every night. In the photo, Lexi is still a pup and Shawn has her in his arms. He is kissing the top of her head as he looks at the camera. This picture allows the boys and him to stay connected. He is thankful that Marie put those photographs in their rooms. Shawn thinks it has helped tremendously in their healing. This way, he knows he is not fading from their memories too quickly.

Then Shawn asked Julie, "Does it get easier to accept over time? I mean, will I ever stop aching for them, and start to feel at peace with the fact I had to leave them?"

Julie replied, "When it is right, and they are ready to move on without you, you will know, and that is when you will have inner peace. It will happen, I promise. While you are guided to acceptance up here, they are on earth discovering their own path of acceptance through people who come in and out of their lives. Their experiences may or may not be fulfilling, but it is all part of the healing. People they had expected to reach out to them will not be able to, while other people, including some they least expect, will be integral to their healing. It is all part of a divine plan."

She continued, "Now, I want to show you something." Julie grabbed Shawn's hand and pulled him to his feet. He followed in silence. The words she spoke were still fresh. He wondered who had been there to help Marie and the boys. He wondered who had reached out to them.

Still lost in his thoughts, he continued to follow blindly along a well-travelled path through the trees and across a bridge over a gently flowing brook.

On the other side of the bridge was a splendid marble archway, and beyond that was the most amazing garden. It was filled with row upon row of asters, dahlias, lilies, and chrysanthemums, intricately interspersed with intense greenery such as hostas, silver queen, dusty miller, and airy grasses. The gardens went on for acre upon acre and appeared to have many different themes. While some sections portrayed a more natural approach with various wildflowers and an organic growing method, other sections followed Asian, tropical, or modernistic themes. He noticed some areas had a cottage feel while others were more contemporary. The fragrant blooms filled his senses. He thought how this must have taken forever to create. This place was simply magical!

It was *poetic* - Julie loved to garden. She had been talented on earth, but this was overwhelming.

"Wow," Shawn said, and he began to weep with happiness. He added, "We all knew you had a purpose in heaven. It was to build your garden! This brings me such joy; I can't even put it into words." Shawn hugged Julie tightly and kissed her head. "You are an amazing girl! Beautiful, just beautiful!"

And they laughed deep belly laughs together, while tears streamed down their cheeks.

Julie saw Romeo coming down the path, and she smiled. He asked, "Can I join you two?"

"Of course you can," they replied simultaneously.

Romeo turned to Shawn, "Isn't this garden amazing? I remember going to visit Julie's and Larry's place when we were on earth. Vivian and I were always impressed with Julie's green thumb. Vivian helps her maintain this place. They stand here for hours talking about annuals and perennials. I have no idea how they can remember the names of all these plants."

Shawn spoke, "Julie and I were having an interesting discussion. Maybe you can shed some light on the subject. There are times we have made our presence known to the people on earth. Have you ever done this?"

Romeo answered, "Yes, as a matter of fact, I was just thinking back to a time I did that very thing. It was about two years after I died and I knew Marie really needed my help, so I sent her a messenger. It was right after she left her first husband and had moved in with her cousin Lorraine for a few weeks."

He continued, "You know how much she loves to swim. Well, one night she needed to clear her head, so she went to the basement where there was a pool and a hot tub. She thought she needed to be alone, but I thought she needed some direction, so I sat in the hot tub and waited. Of course, the messenger didn't look like me, but he was around my age and had a very similar story."

"After she completed her lengths, she entered the hot tub and politely smiled, but tried to send the message that she wanted to be left alone. It took some work, but eventually the messenger got her to talk. His story was very similar to hers. He said he was staying in the building with his daughter because she was going through a rough divorce. He told her he had almost died during triple bypass surgery and he had the scar to prove it. She eventually opened up about her recent separation and told him how she had lost her dad to cancer. At one point in the conversation, I revealed myself briefly, and I saw her face freeze. Then, she shook her head and tried to refocus. There was no mistake; she understood what was going on. I was able to guide her through this very difficult time by coming to her in human form through a messenger."

"She had been down in the pool for almost two hours, and Lorraine was starting to worry, so she came down to see what was taking Marie so long. They met in the stairwell. Lorraine took one look at her and said, 'Are you okay? I was starting to worry.'"

"Marie answered, 'I'm more than okay. I just saw Dad!'"

"'What?'"

"'Yes, he came to me through some other man in the hot tub. I actually saw Dad's face at one point in the conversation, and I thought I was losing my mind. But, then I went to shower on deck and this total stranger put his hand on my shoulder and assured me everything was going to be okay. That wasn't even the weird part,' she said. 'He told me, everything is going to be okay, Marie.'"

"'Yes, and why is that so strange?'"

"'Because, I never told the man my name!' she replied."

Shawn was suddenly overcome with the sense that he needed to be somewhere else...and as he walked away from Julie and Romeo, he realized he was not alone. Raya had returned and she was holding his hand.

It was eight-thirty in the morning and Lexi and Marie were going out for their daily visit to the field. Marie took Lexi off her leash just inside the fence and Lexi broke into a run. Her enormous frame rose and fell with tremendous force – legs leading and skin, muscles, and jowls eventually following, as she pounded the earth. She tore into the ground with her giant paws and one hundred thirty pound frame. Her fawn-coloured coat gleaming in the sunlight, Shawn could see every ripple of muscle move as she beat the ground. She was an incredible force! Her lips gaped open with teeth partially exposed, and her eyes were focused straight ahead with sheer determination. She was a glorious sight! She was *beautiful, powerful, and full of life.*

Shawn watched Marie, as Marie watched Lexi, just marveling in her beauty. He witnessed the stress leaving Marie's body with each breath that entered and escaped her lungs, as her shoulders relaxed. She tilted her face to the sun, closed her eyes, and just lingered in its warm embrace.

And there it was – a connection! They were connected at that moment.

For the first time since his death, he was there with her - both he and Lexi – there for her.

Shawn knew Marie was aware that Lexi was his gift to her. Lexi was that warm body on the bed beside her each night, and when she hugged Lexi, she had hope that she might one day feel whole again.

Then, she thought of the words Shawn had spoken so many times, and he thought of them too, and in perfect unison, they recited the words together.

'Yesterday is History,

Tomorrow a Mystery,

Today is a Gift.

That is why it is called the Present.'

(anonymous)

Chapter Twenty-Five

Our Angel

Lexi was limping and appeared to be favouring her right hip. This was troubling because Lexi was still relatively young, turning three in just a few months.

Having heard that large breed dogs often experience hip dysplasia or joint problems due to the weight they carry while jumping or running, I feared that she was now developing a hip or knee problem. I was keeping a close eye on her to see if the limp would improve or worsen over time.

I had started giving her Glucosamine the year before, was limiting the amount of running she did, and had blocked the stairs in our house to prevent her from jumping on the bed. This was hard to do, because I missed her on the bed and I found it lonely without her body snuggled in tight next to me.

But her limp did get worse and I decided it was time to visit the veterinarian. She hated the vet and immediately went dead weight in the back seat when we pulled up to the door. How do dogs know? Every visit, I literally had to drag her in, or else have someone assist me by pushing from behind. It was quite comical to watch my big tough, guard dog, tail between her legs, trembling in fear.

The vet wasn't certain, but suspected it was her knee, and gave her some Metacam to decrease the pain and inflammation. He instructed me to try this for a week and see if it made a difference. We saw little improvement and returned two weeks later. He suggested we put her under anesthetic and take X-rays to determine the source of her discomfort.

As she was brought into the examination room, her body shook with fear. She shadowed my every move, trying to hide behind me, and then would lean all of her weight into me. I lay down on the blanket beside her while they administered the shot. As I stroked her head and chest, she slowly calmed down and then fell asleep. I didn't want to leave and continued to lay beside her, petting her velvet head and calmly talking to her. When the vet returned, I realized tears were rolling down my face. Lexi meant the world to me and the boys and I couldn't imagine how much harder the last few years would have been without her.

Each hoisting one end of her enormous frame, the vet and his assistant took her into another room, and I went back to the waiting room. After what seemed like an eternity, the vet returned with the results. He told me she would require knee replacement surgery and offered to refer us to a specialist in Edmonton. Then, he informed me that the surgery would cost a minimum of fifteen hundred dollars, depending on the type of surgery we opted to have. The news just got worse, as he added that her other knee may eventually experience the same difficulties, as this is typical of the breed. Of course my mouth dropped open at the price, but how could I refuse? She was only three years old, and I just couldn't imagine life without her! I began to realize we may have purchased a million dollar dog. Yikes! Comically, I thought about the chances of getting Lexi into the movie business, as I had my fortune to regain.

Lexi did have the knee surgery and she recovered extremely well. She was confined to a kennel for the first few weeks and put into a full body harness with two handles on top. We had to use the handles to lift her, to avoid any extra weight on her knee. She looked hilarious: her entire leg was shaved right up to the center of her back, and of course her sad eyes made us melt every time we looked at her.

Considering her young age, I had decided to get Lexi the very best surgery, and just prayed that the other knee would be fine. Her surgery involved a plate instead of wire, which would completely stabilize the knee and give her longevity. The recovery time was nearly two months. We started with short walks, and then slowly progressed to longer walks, and after three long months she seemed good as new.

I made the decision that she would now be limited to leash walks, with no running, to prevent any further injury and to pamper her other knee. But of course, she would get out in the backyard and start ripping around. I would yell at her to slow down and she would stop and turn with a bewildered stare, as if to say, "What's your problem?" and eventually, when she was ready, saunter over to lie down.

The boys doted over her and fiercely protected our baby girl. Cole and Jarryd would lay beside her, stroking her ears... It was impossible not to play with those floppy, velvet ears.

One day, while we were all fussing over her, I looked closely at the marking on her chest and commented to Cole about how much it resembled a white angel with outstretched wings. It was quite amazing we hadn't noticed this before.

From that day forward we called her our angel...and she was, in every way. She gave us comfort in times of sorrow, she gave us joy in times of sadness, and she gave us unconditional love and an unexplainable closeness to Shawn and to God.

This sweet dog carried us through our darkest hours and wrapped us in a blanket of faith which directly led us to spiritual healing. If ever fate came into play, then Lexi was a perfect example; she became the miracle that helped heal us. Even in writing this, my body is filled with tiny electrical impulses, stirring in my chest and branching out to all of my limbs. I feel myself awakening like an angel, as though my body is part of the universe and I have borrowed it for a short while. I am so in awe of the miracles that life has to offer.

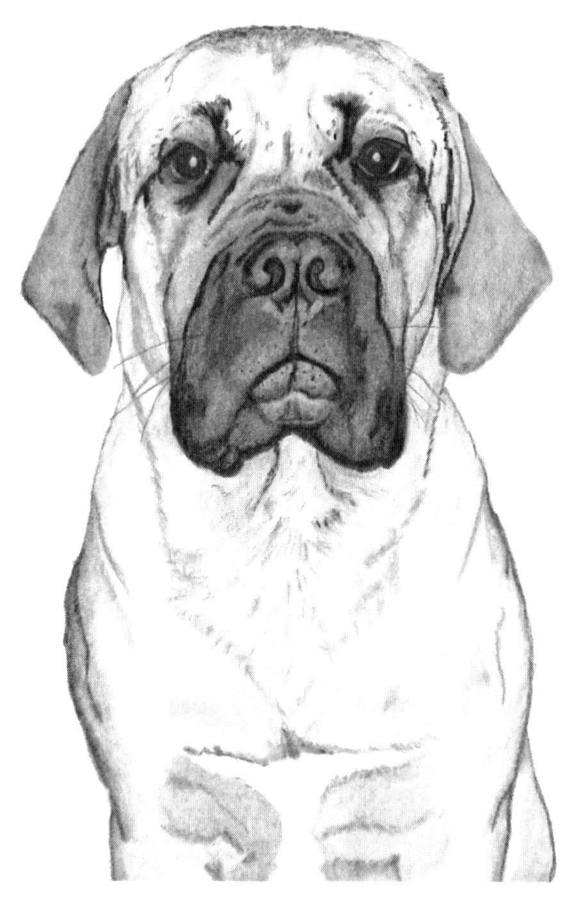

Chapter Twenty-Six

Messages Sent to Heaven

Jarryd and Cole were often late for school the first year after Shawn's death, particularly Cole, who had inherited not only my dad's namesake, but also his unfailing tardiness. Emotions ran high in our house, especially in the mornings. I am not sure why mornings were the worst time, but if I were to venture a guess, it was probably because none of us were getting a restful sleep. Some days we would literally take turns having meltdowns.

At least with the compensation the military had provided, I was able to be there for my boys. I didn't have to rush off to work, and if necessary I could take the whole morning to make sure my boys were settled in school. I thought it extremely important to continue routines, so I spent a lot of time building relationships with the teachers and volunteering in the school. I wanted to make myself available, if the boys ever needed me.

Ms. Kay, the school counselor, was an amazing lady who certainly earned her pay that year. Although she was assigned to my children, some days she would also have me crying in her office. In many ways, she gave all of us strength and held us together. The boys knew that they could ask to leave class if they were having a tough day, and she would always make time for them, if not at that moment, as soon as she was available.

And we were not the only grieving family. There were an unusual number of losses that year. One family had lost their father, another family lost their mother, and the school had also lost one of the teacher aides. The teacher aide was only twenty-one years old and had a rare heart defect.

These losses rocked the school, but if there was a positive in all of this, it was the very strong support group that was put in place. In fact, the school contacted the community health unit who brought in a child psychologist to run something they called the Rainbows Program. This program was designed to bring together all of the students who had suffered a loss, and the objective was twofold: to provide students with healthy coping strategies while allowing them to share their feelings with a peer group.

Ms. Simmons stood next to the pile of coloured paper, instructing the students to choose one piece. Jarryd selected a vibrant blue, knowing this was his dad's favourite colour, while Cole took a soft blue. After each student had made their selection, they went back to the tables and were asked to write messages to the loved ones they had lost.

Then, Ms. Simmons brought each student a helium-filled balloon and asked them to tie their messages to the strings which were already attached to the balloons. Next, she led the students outside to the playground, telling them to hold the strings tightly until they were ready to release their balloons.

When it was time, they watched the beautiful balloons slowly float higher and higher, one-by-one into the sky, eventually making their way beyond the clouds, and out of sight.

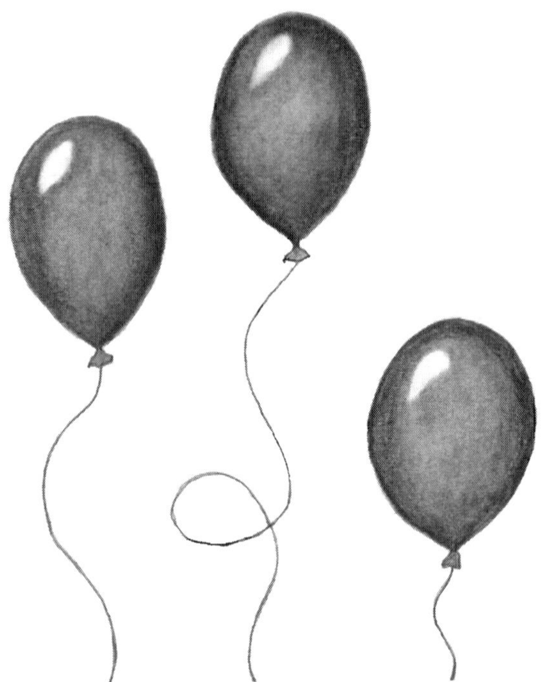

Raya and Shawn watched the children set their balloons free. One young lad stared in amazement; mouth wide, as if wondering if his message could actually reach his mother. A petite girl with auburn hair stood like a statue after she released her balloon, arm still outstretched high above her head, as if by leaving it there she could touch her father's hand.

Shawn saw how Cole tried not to blink, not wanting to miss a moment, but quickly raised his hand and abruptly swiped away the tears that were pooling, letting them roll down his cheeks so he could see again. He didn't move a muscle in his face, as the balloon disappeared forever.

Jarryd simply said a soft prayer, thanking Shawn out loud for being the best daddy in the world!

Shawn squeezed Raya's hand as she pulled him to his feet. He looked up, but could barely see her until his tear streaked vision cleared. The sun was just over the horizon as the balloons started to come into view, with their powerful little notes tied in neat little bows.

For the first time that morning, Shawn realized there were other people standing there with them. It must have been the other parents. He also noticed the young woman they had spoken of who had been cut down in her prime because her heart could not sustain her life. He gratefully acknowledged how he had lived exactly double her age. He was given the opportunity to marry and have children of his own. Suddenly it dawned on him – everyone has their story, some more tragic than others, but ultimately he had to feel lucky for all of the experiences he had lived on earth.

They reached up, giggling like a bunch of children, grabbing hold of the strings that had touched their children's fingers but a few moments before. It was as though their little spirits still lingered there, their beating hearts were still attached, for when they touched the strings they felt a miraculous connection.

They sat in a circle, opening their messages, taking turns reading aloud.

The young woman, Miranda, opened hers first. She had three messages from the three children she had worked with, each expressing how they missed her every day, because she had been the 'bestest' teacher they had ever had. They said they knew she was with God now, in heaven, and this made them happy.

The mother could barely make out the words as she read the messages from her two children. She was choking in tears and her voice broke, wracked with guilt. Shawn surmised from this that she had taken her own life, and her children were saying how she could have shared her unhappiness with them. The last line of her little girl's message had them all weeping: "Daddy loves you and wishes he had hugged you harder that day, so you would have known you were always safe in his arms, where nothing could ever hurt you."

The other father sitting in the circle was also military, but he had died from a roadside bomb while serving overseas. His children wanted to tell him they were okay but that Mommy still cried herself to sleep. But, they said they would continue sleeping with her for as long as she needed them.

Shawn opened Cole's letter.

> *I got your letter Daddy. I am so sorry I said I hated you that day. I never meant it! But Mommy said you know that. Say hi to God and tell him to take care of you. I love you Daddy and we miss you. Xoxoxo*

Shawn laughed a bit through his tears. He put the message down, hoping Cole could hear him, and said, "Cole, I always loved you, no matter what, and I know you didn't mean it son!"

After a few moments, Shawn untied the note from Jarryd.

> *Daddy, I miss our long talks.*
>
> *Mommy tries, but she just doesn't get me! Thank you for all of the things you taught me. I remember how you said Cole and me need to make Mommy laugh every day. We are trying, but it has been hard sometimes. We will try harder. I caught a twenty-one pound salmon and I know you were there. It was the best day ever!*
>
> *I love you Dad.*

Again, Shawn laughed a bit through his tears. He wanted desperately to hold his sons in his arms. In a choked voice, he whispered, "My dear sweet boys. I miss you, my sons."

They sat in that circle most of the morning, sharing stories, and talking about their families. Somehow it made all of them feel better to know that they had a common bond. Who would have ever imagined that you could send messages to heaven.

Chapter Twenty-Seven

Darkest Days

As he walked, the landscape changed from colour to black and white. This place had often crept into his dreams, even though he tried desperately to erase the memories – the destruction of the once picturesque country of Yugoslavia, now lying desolate in a heap of rubble.

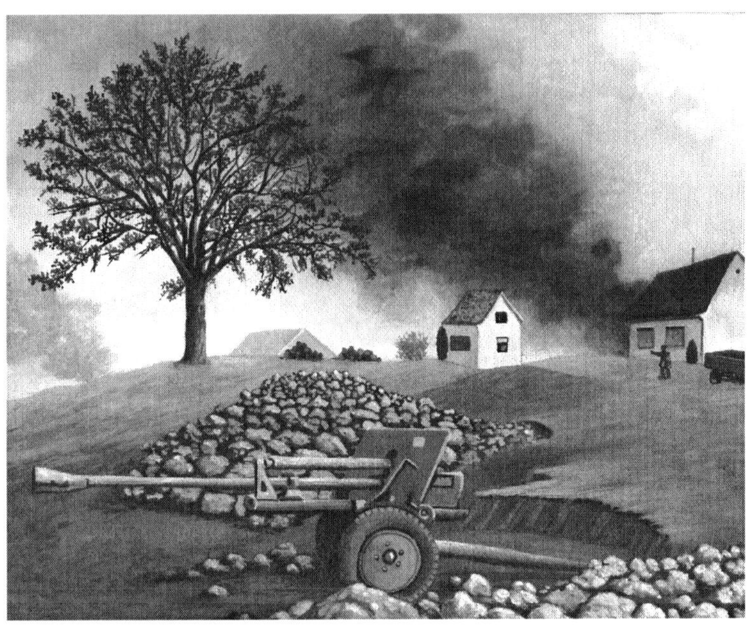

The air was thick with mortar dust. His eyes watered, and his stomach felt as if the contents would surface. But then, his attention was captured by what looked like the silhouette of a young girl emerging from the doorway of a semi-desecrated house. Once his eyes finally adjusted to the greyish haze, he saw that her clothes were filthy and tattered and her frail body staggered in a trance-like state. She froze like a startled, frightened animal when she noticed him approaching, not knowing whether she should stand still, or run. Shawn held his hands out in front of him to show they were empty and he meant her no harm. It was only then that her shoulders relaxed, and she fell to her knees in exhaustion. This place smelled of fear, anguish, and destruction.

This place made him queasy with unforgettable regret.

Seeing the entrance to the house stirred all of his senses. He remembered how it smelled like burnt flesh, and how the mortar dust burned his eyes and the lining of his nose. He felt himself unraveling with fear and horror…remembering the Serbian raids of so many years ago. The year was 1992 and Slobodan Milosevic was in the midst of his tyranny, enforcing genocide on the people of Croatia. Churches, schools, and residences were destroyed based on nationality and religion. If you were lucky enough to be born Serbian and practiced Orthodox Christianity, your life could be spared...but if by fate, you were Croatian, Muslim, or of Roman Catholic faith, your houses and churches were bombed and you would find yourself fleeing, or else experiencing the torturous wrath of the Serbian army. Milosevic was a monster! His objective was to cleanse the land of anyone who did not follow his beliefs, or force them to suffer for their crime of being born of a different race.

Shawn loathed this man. He never understood the stupidity behind racism and the sheer arrogance of considering your people to be a superior race. Are we not all of flesh and blood? The red blood that pulses through our veins and the organs that circulate that blood – are they not identical in every human being?

One day he remembered very well, for it resulted in night sweats for years after, as he relived the peace-keeping missions in his thoughts and dreams. There was one particular memory he desperately tried to erase...

They kicked the door in to find a young girl about the age of nine sprawled across the floor in a bloody mess. Shawn attended to her by immediately checking her vitals. She was still semi-conscious but in a severe stage of shock. One of the other soldiers surveyed the scene and discovered her lifeless father and mother, their hands tied to the backs of the chairs where they sat. Their eyes were fixed in horror, and their heads tilted back to reveal vicious gaping wounds across their necks.

Another soldier went to investigate the putrid smell emanating from the oven. He cautiously approached, fearing what he might find in there, but rather than listen to his better judgment, opened the oven door. Inside, he found a charred roasting pot. The smell of burnt flesh hit him. He removed the pot and lifted the lid. Shawn saw him reel back in utter horror, for in the pot were the burnt remains of a newborn child. That stench would be burned in their memories for all eternity.

He ached with the knowledge that humans were capable of such amoral, barbaric atrocities. What could possibly make someone resort to these actions? To make an innocent little girl and her family suffer such a fate... He felt his heart would explode and he clenched his teeth in venomous hatred. He wanted to tear the savage ruler to bits, piece by piece, and all of the men who followed his command to this end.

Shawn turned his attention to the girl, as he lifted her in his arms and took her outside away from this nightmare. Barely coherent, she nonsensically murmured something in her foreign tongue. He knew her wounds were too deep and there was nothing he could do to help her.

How can man hate with such vengeance? It makes the soul weep! He realized his shirt was drenched, mostly from the sweat that escaped from reliving this hell, but also from the flood of uncontainable tears. All he could do was hold her and sob.

How vicious this cycle of revenge and hatred, always over land and religion. Such petty, petulant greed. Tilting his head to the sky, he let out a cry of anguish that split the heavens. He screamed until his throat was raw, and then fell to his knees, still with the lifeless girl in his arms. At the age of nine, this sweet girl had lost her innocence.

Shawn felt Raya place her hand on his shoulder. He closed his eyes tightly, and finally softened his grasp on the young, lifeless girl.

Raya looked deeply into his eyes and spoke ever so gently, "Shawn, you were not responsible for her death. Forgive yourself for not arriving sooner that day. It was a terrible time to be alive. She is better off. There is no justice for what occurs during any war but God has now provided us with peace. It is time to let the memories go, and to forgive yourself. After all, the sins of man cannot go on destroying us for eternity. It is now your time to heal and to find peace in your heart."

Shawn and Raya walked awhile, hand-in-hand. Raya was silent. Shawn knew that they were both wondering what was wrong with mankind.

Then Raya turned to him and said, "It is my turn to thank you."

"I don't understand," Shawn replied.

"I will forever be indebted to you. Had you not been there that day, my passing would have been unbearable. I was a frightened child, but the moment you arrived, I felt peace. Your heart is pure and your love for mankind is genuine. Shawn, my healing began that day – because of you. From that day forward, I vowed to protect you, like in the car that day, keeping you calm and providing what you needed to survive and carry on in your journey."

Chapter Twenty-Eight

Unbroken Bonds

As Shawn and Raya walked on, the haze began to dissipate and the thick air began to lighten, as did his heart.

Meanwhile, far away in the distance, he noticed a gathering of people. As he moved closer, their individual faces became clear.

He immediately recognized Boomer, one of the first soldiers killed during the Afghanistan mission. Of course, Boomer wasn't his real name, but rather a nickname.

Shawn remembered the day he had watched Boomer's story being broadcast on the evening news, a picture of his smiling face in uniform flashed across the screen. He was only twenty-three. Shawn and Boomer had worked together a few years earlier in Bosnia, and they had remained good friends afterward. One of Shawn's fondest memories of Boomer was in his kitchen on the barracks. Boomer was preparing breakfast for Shawn and a few of the other guys. Being his typical goofy self, he was dancing around, flipping pancakes, and putting on quite the show. They all shared some good laughs. Boomer's spirit was so vivacious!

To see his face on the news… Shawn was crushed, and simply unable to comprehend that he was gone. After all, Boomer was still a kid, with such passion for life and a bright future ahead.

As Shawn approached his friend, both of them teared up, no doubt reliving warm memories. Shawn took Boomer's hand in a handshake and drew him in for a brief, solid hug while slapping his back. "Boomer my man, so good to see you!" Shawn wished he could stay there and have a conversation, but there were so many others to greet. They both knew they would have to save that conversation for another day.

Next to Boomer stood the four soldiers who had lost their lives in the infamous, friendly fire incident in 2002. This was just shortly after the twin towers in New York were attacked on 9/11. Though he had only known one of the soldiers personally, he and Marie had attended the military ceremony at the Coliseum in Edmonton to honour these four men.

He recalled how they had felt like sitting ducks that day, for every dignitary was in that building: the Prime Minister of Canada, the Governor General, the Minister of Defense, the highest ranking military officials, and every available serving member of the forces. The place was filled to capacity (approximately eighteen thousand seats), and with the recent attacks on the United States, the fear was that Canada may be targeted next.

He remembered how Marie had turned to him and asked, "Are you thinking what I'm thinking?"

He had simply squeezed her hand, reassuring her that security was at a maximum. That was true, but they both knew there was always a possibility. He remembered how he had prayed that day, and later breathed a huge sigh of relief when they all stepped safely outside.

These four soldiers stood before him now, and he took turns shaking their hands. He stopped for a moment in front of the soldier he had known.

"Hey man, how did you make it up here?" Shawn asked, grinning ear to ear.

"Yeah, I was thinking the same thing about you, ya old dog!" They exchanged a back slapping guy hug, still chuckling.

From the corner of his eye, Shawn noticed someone repeatedly glancing in his direction, quietly smiling, and waiting patiently for him to finish greeting his military friends. When he took a second look, he couldn't believe his eyes, for there stood his stepfather.

"Ted!" he exclaimed, his voice rising a few octaves. "Oh my God, how wonderful to see you again!"

In that familiar British accent, Ted replied, "Yes lad aren't you the picture? I was wondering when I would set my sights on you again. Ah, let me get a look at ya! My God, you haven't changed a bit! Are they treating you kindly here in heaven?"

"Yes, I've had the grand tour," Shawn replied with a chuckle.

"Ya suppose I could tear you away for a short while so I can chew yer ear a bit, and catch up on what's been happen'n on earth?"

"Yes, certainly Ted, just give me a few moments to get around to everyone. By the way, Ted, have you guys been acquainted? Have you met Boomer, Dyer, and these gentlemen over here?"

Ted replied, "Yes, we've met, but more importantly, we are gathered here to welcome *you!*"

"Really? I'm honoured. So this is the welcome wagon, hey? Aren't you a fine looking group?" Shawn commented with a smile.

Ted had served with the British and later the Canadian military, giving them all a common bond. He had been married to Shawn's mother for over twenty years. Although Ted was not Shawn's biological father, Shawn regarded him as one, stating, "Anyone can father a son, but it takes a certain man to be a father." Ted had always been there for Shawn's mother and had treated her like gold. This was just one of the many reasons Shawn admired and loved this man.

Shawn and his stepfather walked along, catching up on the last five years.

Ted had also battled cancer and was able to relate to what Shawn had gone through. Ted told Shawn how sorry he was that a man of his age had to leave his family behind. "How are those little lads anyway?" he asked.

"They're great, and they keep Marie really busy!"

"I always said enjoy them while they're young. Ah yes, I do remember how they were full of piss and vinegar!"

"Yup, they're busy little boys, always full of energy."

"And how is my Denise? She was there 'til the end ya know? She never left my side. Now thar's a good woman."

"It's been tough for her, Ted. She misses you terribly."

"I never wished to put her though all that. I only wish it had been quick; she was downright exhausted by the end."

"I know," Shawn replied, "but she managed, and she knew you would have done the same for her."

"Ah, you've got that right lad. I would have gone to the end of the world and back for that dear lass. That's for certain! It sure is wonderful to see you, my boy. I have thought of you often."

"There is something I wanted to say to you Ted, but I never got the chance."

"What is it, lad?"

"Thank you for being there for Mom and me. You made her happy. You were like a father to me, and I truly appreciate that."

"Well you know, young fella, I wouldn't have had it any other way."

Shawn continued, "I was thinking the other day about how history repeats itself. My dad's father left him when he was around four years old, then my dad left me when I was four years old, and then I left Amber and Jasmine when they were four and nine years old. I'm not proud of that and I wish I had broken the cycle."

"But you did, with yer own little fellars. You never left them the way your father left you. Your passing was no fault of yer own. Sometimes life deals you a hand and you have to just play your cards and hope for the best. There's no explainin, why some things happen the way they do. You and yer sons had a strong bond. Trust me lad, they'll be okay. Just wait and see! Furthermore, your passing has brought yer girls closer to Marie and the boys as well. It is all a blessing, my dear son."

Chapter Twenty-Nine

Two Years Later

I came across a keepsake box one day while I was cleaning out the basement. In the box, I found all the cards from the funeral wrapped in a huge elastic band. I removed the elastic and began reading the messages that were inside – hundreds of heartfelt sentiments, handwritten by family members and close friends. I vaguely remembered reading them at the time of Shawn's death. Next, I opened the guest book and looked through all of the names listed there. I was stunned. There were so many people I missed seeing that day…or had I? It all seemed like a fuzzy dream.

There was a separate sheet signed by some of the military men and women whom Shawn had been on tour with. I had to laugh at one of the comments in particular:

> *Shawn – you will never be forgotten as my "big brother" who took me under your wing in Bosnia. I will however always blame you for my bad tattoo in Budapest! You will be missed. Rest easy. JoAnne*

Next I began flipping through the pictures. There were various photos of Shawn, the kids, Lexi, and me. I noticed our carefree expressions, and marveled at how the kids had grown and changed over the years.

It felt as though our smiles had been slowly erased…as if the images in the box belonged to someone else's life…like we had been frozen in time.

I continued to reflect back on what seemed a lifetime ago. It took me a moment to cut through the fog and place the images in perspective, reminding myself they had actually been my reality. I thought how the mind plays tricks in order for a person to cope with traumatic experiences. People said I was strong, but I didn't feel strong; I felt numb. Life continued as usual, but the life I once knew stood frozen in time. I would move along in a trance and go through the motions. I remember waiting for my boys in the schoolyard each day after school. Sometimes I would hold back tears when I saw a father interact with his son, yet other times I would simply distance myself…refusing to allow my mind to accept the way things were.

Next, I found a large envelope filled with keepsakes from Shawn. I remembered calling him my 'hearts and flowers' man. After our first date, he had left a single red rose on my doorstep with a note attached, and inside the card was a packet of bath salts. He had remembered! That first night I had told him how I loved to take baths because they seemed to remove all the stress from my life.

This was only the first of many flowers, cards, sticky notes, postcards, letters, and poems, always with his illustrated heart with an arrow through it…

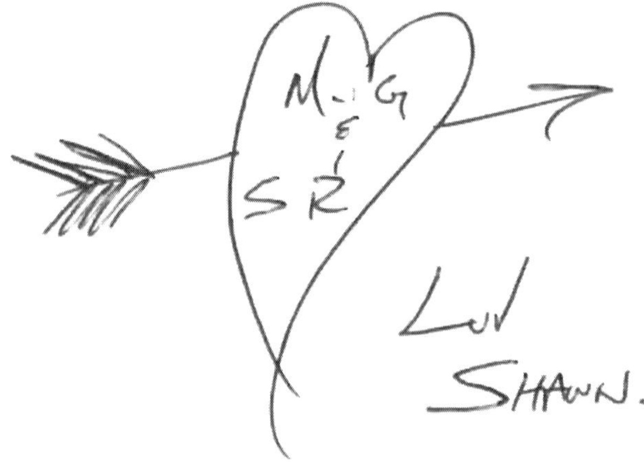

Not a day went by that he didn't say "I love you." I still have a small stone carving he gave me, embedded with two dolphins. He bought it on a trip and attached this poem. He wrote the poem while on the plane flying home, and then he carefully cut the words into a paper heart:

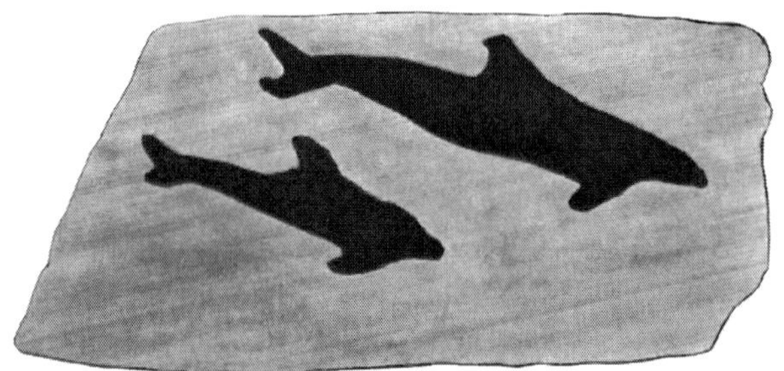

To The Love of My Life,

This carving symbolizes our love.
At first it was large
But, in time like our lives
Certain parts required to go elsewhere.
To which God slowly removed surface features
Thus, two figures remain in stone for all time.

Our love shall remain solid like dolphins who
Live with one mate eternally.
Look deep into the carving and see
How we gracefully and patiently
Move through the water like life.
Look deep into my eyes
For they will show you
My love is eternal.

Marie, my heart, body and soul
are yours eternally
Love forever
Shawn

He was a true romantic. We made a point of going on a date at least once a month, and continued even after the kids were born. I got this idea from a secretary at the school where I worked. She was in her late fifties and I had noticed how she and her husband had kept their romance alive after more than thirty years of marriage. One day I had asked her for their secret. She explained: a couple still needs to find ways to connect, even after they have children. She said this may mean locking the bathroom door and having a bubble bath together, going for a romantic dinner and movie, or maybe just a simple walk, as long as you always find ways to share your love. That way, when the kids are gone, you will still know the person who you married. It takes effort, because the kids can take up all of your time and energy if you let them. Too many couples discover that once the children leave, they find themselves staring at a stranger.

This was awesome advice!

Chapter Thirty

Time to Live Again

It was fall of 2010, and I felt it was time to start living again. It was as though I had emerged from behind a heavy black curtain. Suddenly, I wanted to travel, to spend more time with family, to share every possible experience with my boys, and to feel alive! I booked a trip to Florida so that the boys could meet the cousins on their dad's side of the family and also visit their half-sisters Jasmine and Amber. It became clear to me how important it was to stay in contact with family. A few months later, we traveled to California. I took Jarryd and Cole to Disneyland and we stayed with relatives from my side of the family.

I applied to work as a substitute teacher with my previous employer. My boys couldn't be happier that Mom was teaching again. In fact, they loved when I taught in their classrooms. I thought they would be creeped out in front of their peers, but strangely, they always beamed with pride, telling me I was the best teacher in the world. (Of course, I paid them to say that!)

As I stood in front of my students, I felt a renewed confidence. There is something to be said about being a survivor. As tough as life has been at times, I persevered. Yes, I made plenty of mistakes along the way, but at least I learned from them. I thought if I could teach my children anything, it would be how to survive – to be able to laugh and realize all people make mistakes. Most of all, I wanted them to work hard to achieve their dreams.

Shawn was living proof of that. I will always use him as an example of someone who never gave up and never stopped living every day as though it were his last. It was as though he had his own private bucket list of things to accomplish, and never stopped checking off those items. I hope he has no regrets for the way he lived his life. I know how proud he made his family and all the people who knew him.

As I gained this new confidence, I remembered how he had told me I would have to go on one day, and eventually open myself up to the possibility of finding love again. I figured if it happened, it happened, but my kids would always be my main focus. Those two young boys needed me and I would do everything in my power to give them every opportunity life had to offer.

This is not to say life was easy. We had our fair share of difficult times. I had two extremely bullheaded, passionate boys, and I was now a single Mom.

I'm still not sure where they got their stubbornness from – must have been their father!

I had a lot of work to do and the battle to steer us in the right direction seemed unreachable at times. Even so, we needed to get on with life. As my mother used to say, "The pity party was over." Brutal as this was, it was true. Hard as it was, there was nothing we could do to change what we had gone through. Certainly, we still had our moments of weakness, and we took time to comfort each other, but our grief could no longer stifle our hopes and dreams. After all, would Shawn have wanted us moping around – or would he have told us to smarten up, to enjoy life and all it has to offer? I think we all know the answer to this…

Eventually, I went on a few dates, but certainly not with the expectation of finding love again. Then I met Ray – adorable Ray with a Ukrainian background and a great sense of humour. We met for lunch on our first date, and on our second date we met for dinner and a movie. This is when I explained I had two very precocious, vivacious boys at home and told him he would be wise to 'RUN!' But the foolish guy stayed. I figured he had been fairly warned, so we continued to date. I just felt safe with him right from the beginning. When Lexi approved, I knew he was okay.

Lexi had always cowered around men she didn't know. I'm not certain if that was simply her nature, or if something had happened when she was a pup to make her afraid. She had to warm up to men, yet she would instantly go to any woman or child. It was actually comical to see this big wuss hiding behind me whenever a man would approach. I often wondered if she would actually protect me if I was ever 'really' in trouble, and I have to confess, I had my doubts! But with Ray, it only took a few minutes before she went over and began licking his face. Mind you, he had a treat in his hand, but still, this was a first for her.

Ray connected with the boys right away, even though he didn't have any children of his own. He had been married before, but he and his ex-wife had made the choice not to have children. Being the youngest of a large family, Ray had plenty of experience with his numerous nieces and nephews. It was instantly clear: he was a natural with children. The most endearing quality was his down to earth attitude and ability to be a 'big kid' himself. By the way he interacted with Jarryd and CoIe, I knew he had been raised in a loving family, with strong morals and values.

Soon, we were introduced to Georgia, Ray's Malamute-Golden Retriever cross. She was a beautiful dog. She fit in very well, unless it was feeding time. Lexi learned the hard way not to interfere while Georgia was eating. I believe it may have had something to do with being an 'only child'.

The first time the fighting at mealtime happened, the kids were screaming and crying, keeping their distance from the dogs, and cowering on the couch. Georgia had grabbed Lexi by the lip and she would not let go! Lexi was shaking and just standing there like a dummy. With her size, she could have easily defended herself, but I think dogs have a hierarchy and the older ones get the respect regardless of their size. I grabbed Georgia by her collar and dragged her to the floor, scolding her.

Jarryd was bawling and Cole was screaming.

When the boys reacted the way they did, Ray thought I would send him and his dog packing. He knew the story of how Jarryd had been mauled and understood how fearful the boys must have been. After that day, the dogs were fed separately. Georgia and Lexi became good companions. They loved their walks together, and Lexi liked having a buddy to hang out with when the humans were away. Eventually we relaxed our feeding habits, but the same thing happened again.

Although Georgia was never aggressive with people, she had a history of going after other dogs. I told Ray I couldn't take the chance of it being the boys she turned on the next time. He was reluctant, but in complete agreement.

Georgia was nearly twelve years old and had fairly severe arthritis in her hips, which may be why she had become so crotchety. Ray made the difficult decision to have her put down. He loved that dog and we knew how hard this was for him. Ray cremated Georgia and scattered her ashes along the trails where they had frequently walked in the river valley.

Ray lost his oldest brother Jim one year later. The horrible "C" word had stolen yet another loved one from us. This served as yet another reminder of how precious life was. The four of us began to travel, taking numerous trips all over Canada, U.S.A., and Mexico. We purchased a travel trailer and spent most of our summers camping and fishing. We even took scuba lessons.

I sensed Shawn smiling down on us, taking comfort in knowing the boys and I were in good hands.

Life was good!

Chapter Thirty-One

Just Breathe

Nothing but water above me…in pitch blackness.

My mask had been blacked out, designed to simulate a 'dead flashlight' on a night dive. I began to panic, feeling completely out of my comfort zone, and threw off my weight belt and my body immediately ascended to the surface.

I was desperate. I felt I needed to get my face to the surface, to take in real air and remove this dark, claustrophobic mask from my face. I was overcome with genuine fear. Fear of what, I wasn't certain. My life was not in danger. I was still breathing through my air regulator.

I ripped off the mask which allowed me to see again and the relief was instantaneous…but now I realized I was completely screwed, because my body is extremely buoyant. I can float as effortlessly as a baby seal; ask me to sink to the bottom though and watch the thrashing begin! In fact, the instructor had provided a heavier weight belt just so I could reach the bottom.

I was done for. I would definitely fail the course.

The instructor tried to calm me, and then challenged me to think outside the box. He just kept repeating, "Complete the task." I was getting really annoyed with him.

"How do I get to the bottom without my weight belt?" I asked haughtily.

"Deflate your lungs."

He was challenging me to think, and I wanted to scream!

He suggested, "Blow all the air out of your lungs and swim to the bottom."

With an exasperated sigh, I donned my blackened mask again, blew all of the air I possibly could out of my body, and swam like hell for the bottom. It worked! I was able to finally retrieve the weight belt from the bottom of the dive tank.

Next, came the struggle to strap it around my waist. The thick thermal dive gloves which restricted my sense of touch and dexterity made this task even more difficult. All the while, I reminded myself, "*Just breathe, Marie.*"

I hated the sensation of being unable to see, but desperately wanted to complete this task because I knew the swimming would be a piece of cake. My fingers clumsily fumbled, desperately trying to feel the edges of the buckle… I thought I would be home free if I could just locate the buckle's opening and slide the loose end of the belt through. But the belt started to present more difficulty as I had it all twisted about. Soon, I found myself thrashing from side to side, cursing in my head and praying that I catch a break.

"Why couldn't I catch a break!? Why couldn't the hole in the buckle miraculously present itself?"

Meanwhile, the only sound was the air entering and escaping the breathing apparatus, simulating a very agitated 'Darth Vader'. Panic was beginning to set in. I wanted to let a few choice words rip, but I couldn't speak with the ventilator in my mouth. My mind swarmed in every direction and my breathing got even quicker. Then I realized I wasn't fighting for air. I had air. What I desperately wanted to escape was the vulnerability I felt. This was familiar territory...the lack of control over my life…it was all bullshit, quite frankly, and I thought about quitting and storming away in defeat. But hadn't I already quit too many times? Hadn't I given up, thinking it was just too hard; like when I had bailed one hundred feet from the top of Middle Sister Mountain? My life was not in jeopardy at this moment, but my pride sure was. Giving up now would be like surrendering to every bad thing that had ever happened in my life. So I fought, first letting my body go limp, releasing my fear and then letting every muscle in my body relax.

Hot tears were streaking my face, but then the most amazing thing occurred. I stopped struggling, and conceded to my fears – these demons that represented every abominable thing that had occurred over these past five years – I surrendered to all of it and realized I couldn't quit. I thought, "I'll be damned if I am going to let this defeat me!"

Then, I remembered the instructor's last words: "Focus on your breathing...controlled breaths in and out...as long as you have air, you are going to be okay."

I thought with acknowledgement and gratitude, "Isn't that the truth. When life presents challenges and kicks you down-*just keep breathing*."

Epilogue

On August twelfth, 2019, marking the eleventh anniversary of their father's death, Jarryd and Cole tackled the arduous hike up Middle Sister Mountain. It seemed a lifetime ago.

Mom had prepped them, ensuring they were carrying enough water and snacks to sustain their strength.

As Jarryd followed Cole across the lower plateau of dense bush, he decided it was time to have a little fun. "Watch out for bears, Cole!" he warned.

Cole, slowing his steps, walked a little more cautiously.

Jarryd continued to unnerve him. "Remember how Dad said he encountered a bear here at the bottom?"

Cole, growing more agitated, instinctively swung his arm back, hoping to strike some part of Jarryd's body. But, Jarryd anticipated this reaction and leapt back a few steps.

Jarryd continued, "Dad said he had been making his way through the dense bushes along a trail like this and the trees were loaded with red, juicy berries, ripe for the picking. Then, as he stepped into the next clearing, and without any warning, he came upon a black bear cub feasting on the berries. He froze in his tracks, but soon his gaze landed on the bushes just a few feet behind the cub. There was mama bear! She stood six feet tall! Dad's first instinct had been to run, but he quickly reconsidered, and cautiously retraced his steps backward, one foot behind the other…careful not to make a sound. Once he was out of sight, he hauled ass to a safe clearing. He told Mom it was a frightening experience. He said he had been paralyzed with fear, but still remembered all of the correct things he needed to do. He knew that if he had panicked, even for a moment, he would have quickly become prey and if the mama bear had sensed her cub was threatened, he was good as dead."

Cole said, "Shut up and hike. You're freaking me out!"

Jarryd giggled.

After checking his watch, Jarryd discovered that the climb had taken four hours. The spectacular Canadian Rockies were laid out for miles in every direction. He and Cole were now able to fully appreciate the story Mom had recounted about the difficult climb. As they stood at the peak, they understood why Dad had longed to reach the summit. In their eighteen and twenty years on earth, they had never encountered anything so breathtaking. The view was spectacular – everything they had imagined!

Jarryd raised his arms high above his head, feeling the rush of the wind as it grabbed and tussled his hair in every direction. He closed his eyes for a moment, which gave him the sensation of floating above the earth.

Cole couldn't resist, and followed his brother's lead.

They laughed like children, screaming out, "I'm King of the world! *I'm King of the world…*"

"Hello…*hello…hello…*"

Their words echoed from the mountain top, bouncing off the rocks-disappearing in the great expanse.

Jarryd retrieved the two small urns from his backpack and handed one to Cole.

Jarryd twisted the cap off the urn which contained his father's ashes. He explained, "Daddy, Lexi was always meant to be your dog. We knew it was your plan, to have her protect us on Earth. She gave us the best years of her life and provided us with the comfort in knowing you were always with us. Now, she is yours again and will remain with you for all eternity. We know she will give you as much joy as she brought into our lives. We will miss our little angel," a lump now formed in his throat, "but we're at peace knowing she is with you."

Cole removed the cap on the urn which contained Lexi's ashes. Tears streaked his face as he said, "Lexi, we are sending you home to be with your master. May you and Dad run like the wind in heaven. Tear up the earth, my sweet girl, and give Daddy those big sloppy kisses. Make sure he knows that many of them are from his boys."

Standing shoulder to shoulder, Jarryd and Cole tilted the urns just enough to allow the wind to catch the ashes. As the ashes lifted off the mountain top, they began to dance and intermingle as one…

In Heaven

Shawn heard heavy footsteps off in the distance… A thousand tiny pin pricks electrified his body. Over the hill he saw her, and thought he must be dreaming.

Her enormous frame rose and fell with tremendous force – legs leading with skin, muscles, and jowls eventually following, as she pounded the earth. She tore into the ground with her giant paws and one hundred and thirty pound frame. Her fawn coat gleamed in the sunlight and he could see every ripple of muscle move as she beat the ground. She was an incredible force! Her lips gaped open with teeth partially exposed, and her eyes focused straight ahead with sheer determination. What a sight to behold! Seeing her, Shawn felt like a ten year old boy again. She was beautiful, powerful, and full of life!

His face was soaked with tears of joy. She was his dog now. He had been waiting for her.

Acknowledgements

I am ever grateful to our family and friends for the love and unlimited support we received during this time. It is impossible to mention every person; therefore, I apologize in advance if I have missed anyone. It was my hope to weave the story around all of the individuals who touched our lives, but there were just too many.

First, I would like to thank everyone who came to visit Shawn at the hospital and in our home in Ottawa. Also, I am thankful for all who visited him in Edmonton, especially those of you who travelled great distances to lend your support.

A special thanks to every military member who stepped in to help, especially the group of soldiers who built Lexi a custom dog house complete with siding, shingles, and a name plate; and the troops who helped us relocate in Fort Saskatchewan.

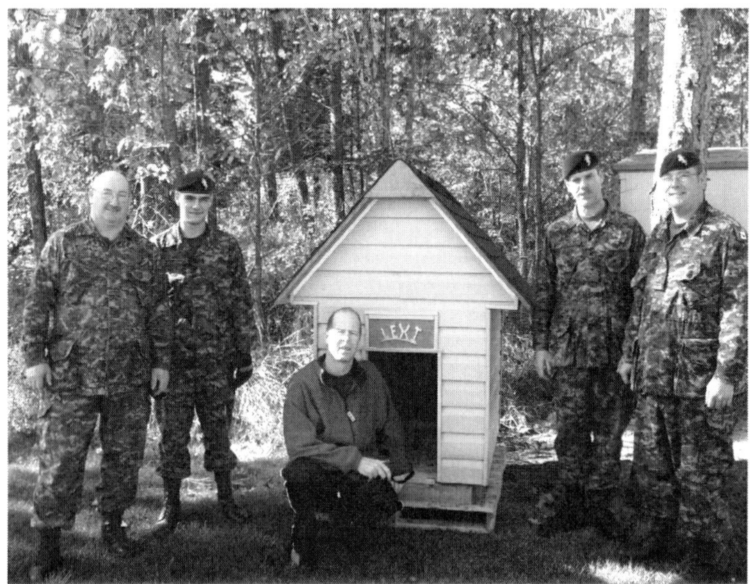

I will never forget Corporal Wanda Lowen, who appeared in our lives once we were posted back to CFB Edmonton. She was assigned to us through the military to take care of paperwork and ensure that everyone had the necessary transportation and documentation, but she became so much more than that. She took the role of pseudo-Grandmother for Jasmine, Amber, Jarryd, and Cole, and reached out to me as a friend. She opened up her house to us all and provided emotional support and nurturing. This was not part of her job, but purely out of the kindness of her heart. I will always love her for taking care of us.

Also, I thank Sergeant Kevin Dickson, my supporting officer and dear friend. He knew how to remain calm and supportive every step of the way, but also knew how to make me laugh when I wanted to cry.

Shawn's dear friend Richard Groten, who flew to Ontario to visit, bringing with him one of the most precious gifts Shawn ever received: a small glass container filled with gravel from the mountain-biking trails where he and Shawn spent many hours riding. Richard's one small gesture brought Shawn newfound hope and incredible joy.

My cousin Lorraine, who without fail, was first on the scene to rescue me and provide emotional support.

My friend Shelly, who was at the hospital almost every day to provide love and spiritual support.

My neighbours Rosemary and Dave, who rescued me and the boys several times after Shawn passed, and renewed my faith in God's love. Also, our dear friends Sandy and Norbert, for their endless friendship and support.

My friend Annette, who grew up with brothers and always knew how to make Shawn laugh with her sassy comments.

Michelle, Bruce, Kassandra, Spensor, Jarred, Pierse, and Quentin, who were there for us when we needed love, support, and family.

Lisa and Brian Hoban, for the incredibly therapeutic retreats to the beach house and for the love they give effortlessly every day of their lives; as well as Aunt Sherron, Uncle Alan, Jenny, and Joann who took the boys and me under their wings, loving and protecting us as only they could do.

Also, Nathalie who Shawn loved as a sister. Thank you for your visit to Ottawa while Shawn was in radiation treatments. This was an extremely difficult time and to see your beautiful, smiling face, gave Shawn the strength and encouragement he needed.

Dennis and Kathy, Marcel and Kathy, and all of our cousins in California who opened up their homes to the boys and me. We had an amazing time reconnecting with all of you; your faith, love and support will always be remembered.

Victor and Kirsten Jordan and family, for the trip to the Island and the beautiful colour photo album which marks these amazing memories.

Eric, Shawn's lifelong friend, who never once missed calling him on his birthday, and who travelled from Toronto to give Shawn support while he was in the hospital. Also, Richard Creamer, Shawn's cousin whom Shawn loved as a brother, always holding him in the highest regard. Richard was always there for Shawn as they shared a remarkable friendship and eternal bond.

Mark, Norman, Janice, and Suzanne who jumped on the next plane to Ontario when I said I needed them.

Also, all of the wonderful friends we made while living in Pembroke, and the many great poker nights.

A special thanks to Phyllis, who became instrumental in completing this novel. I had been struggling with it for months, and she, having gone through something very similar with her husband, was committed to helping me finish. She was a fresh pair of eyes and for the most part objective, as she knew very little about my story.

Rae Anne, my dear friend since grade school, who is responsible for the beautiful illustrations and artwork throughout the novel.

My dear friend Stephanie who edited the final proof. She helped to bring my voice to life, and carry forth the powerful messages in this book.

Denise, for her love and endless strength through all of this. And, on Denise's behalf, I would like to thank her family, who travelled across Canada to support her. I could see how her shoulders instantly relaxed, as she felt the comfort of her siblings and extended family around her.

Jasmine and Amber who travelled from Florida to spend the final month with their dad. This meant the world to him. Please always remember how proud he is of you both! Furthermore, words cannot express how much having you there for support meant to Nana, the boys, and me.

Ray, for encouraging me to finish, often helping me find the words, and always believing in me with his endless love and encouragement.